Lazar Beinin

Medical Consequences of Natural Disasters

With 45 Figures and 40 Tables

Springer Verlag
Berlin Heidelberg New York Tokyo

Dr. med. Lazar Beinin
Rehov Hamorad 8/8
17000 Nazareth/Ilit, Israel

ISBN-13: 978-3-540-15506-5 e-ISBN-13: 978-3-642-70532-8
DOI: 10.1007/978-3-642-70532-8

Library of Congress Cataloging in Publication Data. Beinin, L. (Lazar), 1915–. Medical consequences of natural disasters. Bibliography: p. 1. Natural disasters – Hygienic aspects. 2. Emergency medical services. 3. Disaster relief. 4. Disaster medicine. I. Title. [DNLM: 1. Disaster Planning. 2. Disasters. 3. Emergencies. 4. Emergency Medical Services. WB 105 B422m] RA645.9.B45 1985 362.1'8 85–8141

2119/3140-543210

For my wife Polina

Preface

In spite of all the progress made by modern science and technology in penetrating the mysteries of nature and providing new possibilities for its transformation, we remain largely helpless in the face of such natural phenomena as earthquakes, tsunami, typhoons, floods, and droughts. Natural disasters occur suddenly, but with periodicity, and man has been confronted by their devastating consequences throughout history.

The way people deal with these problems is primarily predetermined: by character, by conditions, and by the social and economic development of society. Industrious efforts to reconstruct nature, and exploitation of her resources, have brought about additional damage, and there is the apparent danger that our interference with the atmosphere and other areas such as climate, soil, and hydrology has initiated devastating processes which may well be irreversible. As a result, the effects of natural disasters, and all the ensuing repercussions, become ever more aggravating. Their scope becomes global, and for the time being we have no effective countermeasures at our disposal with which to fight them.

The contemporary world, then, faces the interconnected and interdependent phenomena of ecological crises and natural disasters: the problem of protecting man from the environment, and the concurrent problem of protecting the environment from man.

We are concerned here with medical ecology, which is obviously ethically grounded, in its study and analysis of modern life. An important example is the intensive development of transport capacities, accompanied by massive road traffic catastrophes involving deaths and injuries – for natural disasters are determined both by natural factors and by man's activities.

The devastation that follows directly affects the environment, people's health and way of life, and the economy.

In the ensuing emergency situation – after man has fallen from the heights of civilization created by his own genius – there is a desperate need for highly effective health services and social stability. The readiness of the public health services and the responsiveness of a society under stress are tested to the limits. Sanitary, hygienic, and everyday domestic conditions are intensified to the point of bursting by epidemic processes. Frequently, information is abnormally received and interpreted. Injured people and those around them tend to become demoralized. One of the problems is a rise in crime, and the danger of anarchy and its accompanying phenomena is especially acute.

People accustomed to the amenities of contemporary life suffer greatly when deprived of them by natural disasters. The suffering is especially unbearable when several natural disasters strike a region simultaneously, leaving the population helplessly facing new and extreme conditions.

Disasters frequently take on cataclysmic proportions. The regular rhythm of life is paralyzed. An area cannot solve its problems without outside assistance, owing to a discrepancy between the medical needs of the injured and the objective capabilities of the local medical services.

There is enough evidence testifying to the readiness of other countries to provide necessary help. However, practical deployment of resources based on a rationally elaborated plan must include:

a) the organization of emergency teams especially for this purpose, equipped to provide medical and other aid, and the determination of their operational activities, and
b) assessment of the requirements for and the delivery and distribution of food, clothing and medicine, and temporary accommodation for those made homeless.

In a sense, the organization of emergency measures under disaster conditions and the ability to cope with the problems arising, including jeopardized public health and safety, may serve as an index of a country's social and economic foundations and of its civil defense preparedness. Experience in fighting natural disasters has shown an almost universal lack of preparedness in providing effective, wellorganized help to the injured and the stricken area. Many lives are lost, health is endangered, and material damages are huge. Nonetheless, the tendency to remain inactive, to prefer risk to preventive measures (which require considerable expenditure and are therefore generally unpopular) appears to prevail at all levels of decision-making.

Preventive measures are here understood as actions relevant to the long term, and preference is given to solving problems which appear more immediate. Consequently, there is a tendency to postpone preliminary elaboration and implementation of the following aspects of an interconnected and interrelated relief system:

1. Complex preventive and defensive measures must be implemented in handling the effects of ecological crisis, earthquakes, tsunami, and droughts. Anthropogenic disasters such as road traffic catastrophes must also be taken into account
2. Help must reach the focus of the disaster in the shortest possible time, rescue operations must be launched immediately, and medical and other aid must be provided
3. Comprehensive information on the scope and intensity of the disaster must be collected and processed, and the activities of the various health authorities responsible for ameliorating the situation must be coordinated

This volume addresses the following medical consequences of natural disasters:
1. Effects on public health and safety
2. Peculiarities of the emergency situation; the main natural and other factors predetermining the organization of medical aid and the evacuation of the homeless

3. Provisions for public health and safety in the event of disaster, and sanitation of the environment

Known natural disasters are investigated, with emphasis placed on the natural, socioeconomic, and other factors affecting the areas and the populations stricken. Among others, the following events are discussed:

1. Earthquakes in Japan (1923), the Crimea (1927), Tajikistan (1930), Armenia (1934), Moldavia Soviet Socialist Republic (1940), Ashkhabad (1948), Tashkent (1966), and Guatemala (1976)
2. Tsunami in Japan (1896), Italy (1908), the Hawaiian Islands (1946), the USSR (1952, 1960), Chile (1960), and Bangladesh and India (1970)
3. Floods in the USSR (1914, 1924, 1964, 1966, 1969)
4. Mudflows and snowslides in the USSR (1921, 1963, 1967), England (1966), and Peru (1970)
5. Mass hunger in the USSR (1921–1922), Leningrad under blockade (1941–1942) and western Africa (1973)
6. Road traffic catastrophes in Israel

Analysis of the ensuing injuries and of infectious and general diseases is based mainly on documentary data of the USSR public health authorities and on the literature from other countries.

The material and its analysis are treated here in light of my personal experience in combating and taking preventive measures against the public health consequences of natural disasters (Moldavia, 1940; Kamchatka, 1957, 1960). Special trips made to stricken areas – Greece, Italy, Russia, the Ukraine, and the United States – facilitated deeper understanding of the situations and, to a certain extent, concrete evaluation of future prospects. Experience in the field of health services as organized in Central Asia and my military experience in World War II have been used as well.

Drawing, then, on more that four decades of firsthand experience of natural disasters in many different countries, I find that some general observations can be made. For example, it is not only that the danger is often underestimated. Frequently, socioeconomic, political, and administrative difficulties obstruct mobilization of the considerable resources needed for efficient prophylaxis and protection, even though, objectively speaking, all the necessary material and technology are at the disposal of those responsible for dealing with these problems. Obviously, natural disasters cannot be prevented. However, damage and lives lost can be kept to a minimum through a proper application by man of his knowledge and technology. I hope that the present study will help to further this end.

Nazareth, May 1985 L. Beinin

Contents

A Brief Historical Review of Natural Disasters

For all its importance and immediacy, the problem of natural disasters remain unsolved. On the one hand, it involves protecting man from nature; on the other, in light of observed ecological crises, it frequently involves protecting nature from man. Excessive activity toward a more efficient use of nature, and toward its reformation, can lead to anthropogenic natural disasters.

In his treatment of nature, in reevaluating his attitude to nature, and in his endeavor to reach *infinita potestas*, man has become highly inventive, though not very wise. In a sense, while he is freer of the elemental forces of nature, man now finds himself controlled by his own technology and the new living conditions that it has created. This process is irreversible. Under certain circumstances, when the ecology of an environment is disturbed, things may get seriously out of control, and as the Austrian scientist, Heimer, concluded, the need arises for a new scientific field, that of anthropogeology, to study the impact of man's activity on various aspects of nature.

Since ancient times, man has observed the devastating and depressing effects of natural disasters. He struggles against them, always unsuccessfully, his desperately contrived means of protection never effective enough. Passive acceptance of his lot always predominated over useful activity. The basic reason for passivity was lack of knowledge and insufficient material means. Towns and settlements have been destroyed, countries brought to ruin.

The social significance of the public health consequences of natural disasters are tremendous, as can be determined by the magnitude of damages, indiscriminately affecting all segments of the population, and by the migration of large groups of people and its consequent impact on the social, economic, and political conditions of the area, as well as on the defensive potential of a country in a purely military sense.

The earthquake in Judaea, which happened during the time of Herod (101 years before the destruction of the Second Temple) took 30 000 lives. This event made enemy invasion easy, having brought about a desperate loss of self-control among the Jews (Josephus Flavius [80]). Though belonging to the ancient past, this tragedy sounds quite immediate today, and serves as an illustration of an existing possibility. Throughout history, large communities and whole countries have suffered the consequences of natural disasters. These events may serve as valuable analogues for a methodology today.

Considering the problem of forecasting earthquakes, Gorshkov [104] states: "If it is known that a certain natural calamity took place under certain conditions and was accompanied by a certain development of events, it may be presumed that the same circumstances, the same combination of conditions can bring about similar calamities."

In the earthquake in Antioch (526 AD), 260 000 people were killed. In 2 min in Calabria (1783), an earthquake ruined 109 towns and villages. Of a population of 166 000, 32 000 (19.3%) were lost [170]. The earthquake in China in 1556 brought about a huge landslide; the number of victims reached about a million [215]. In India a devastating calamity took place on October 7, 1732. A tidal wave came into the Bay of Bengal, taking 300 000 lives and destroying 20 000 ships [39]. India and Bangladesh have been struck by similar disasters right up to the present day.

As is generally known, earthquakes and submarine volcanic eruptions are closely connected with tsunami. Since 687 AD, of 99 recorded tsunami on the Japanese Islands, 17 have caused catastrophic damage. On July 15, 1896, tsunami attacked northwest Honshu and southern Hokkaido in seven gigantic waves covering a coastline of about 300 km, killing 27 000 people and washing away or destroying 10 000 buildings.

The catastrophic tsunami of August 27, 1883 was the direct result of a volcanic eruption (Krakatoa). After the strongest submarine explosion, huge waves lashed the island of Java. At certain points the waves reached a height of 36 m. The coastal towns of Anjer, Bentam, Merak, and others (in the northwest part of Java and on the banks of the Sibezi) were destroyed. About 40 000 people were killed. Another such outburst could occur in the same region; it seems only a question of time. Research is therefore being carried out to determine the possibility of predicting such a calamity.

Periodically occuring floods and mudflows have been reported since ancient times, with especially devastating consequences. The Ganges flood in 1864 took 48 000 lives; another flood in 1876 (the Brahmaputra River) killed 200 000. The Yangtze River flood in China in 1931 swept 140 000 to their deaths. Periodic floods in these areas are no less damaging today. In 1966, flooding of the Ganges, the Brahmaputra, and the Meghna rivers and their tributaries sank an area tens of thousands of square kilometers in India. Thirteen million people resided in this area; tens of thousands of houses were destroyed and a great many people were killed [275]. What was unexpected in this case was the timing, not the possibility of the disaster. Neither can the scope of the damage caused by the flood and its direct consequences be considered unexpected. Nonetheless, organization of appropriate preventive and protective measures was clearly lacking. This experience showed that the expenses for organization and implementation of such measures would have been far less than what was in fact paid for the consequences.

Another aspect to consider when evaluating the damages caused by natural disasters is hunger. Hunger is caused by both floods and droughts.

Between 206 BC and 1911, China suffered 3106 floods and 1873 droughts. In 1828 cases, mass hunger was reported. The universally known famine in Bangladesh (1974) was the direct result of a flooding of the Brahmaputra.

Rousseau [215] describes the consequences of the Messina earthquake (1908) as an instance of man's light-minded attitude toward natural disasters. The earthquake was quite moderate, but because of the lack of any activity on the part of the authorities, there was severe damage, and 160 000 lives were lost.

Mankind prefers to study errors committed in the past: Strong earthquakes supply material for subsequent research activities; every new calamity is a lesson, providing researchers with new facts. In China in 1920, a catastrophic earthquake affected an area of 150 000–450 000 km^2. Two hundred thousand people died. The majority of the deaths in this case were due to the effects of loess [248].

Especially instructive for researchers was the Kwant earthquake, which occured on September 1, 1923 (also known as the Tokyo, or Yokohama earthquake). Its magnitude was 8.2 on the Richter scale. According to the press, the earthquake affected five towns and ten provinces with a total population of nine million. In 60 s, 50–80% of all houses in the cities and towns were destroyed. In Tokyo city alone, 1.5 million people were made homeless; in the whole Tokyo prefecture this figure reached 1.8 million. During a 2-week period (September 2–16) about 3 170 000 people left the capital. Fire broke out after the earthquake and lasted for three days. The temperature in the city rose from the normal 25°–26° C to 46° C. Three-fourths of the residential area was reduced to ashes. Helpless victims escaped to higher-lying parts of the city, public places, and parks. Over 40 000 gathered in the Military Clothing Depot Square; 38 000 were burned to death. According to the official report issued in 1926, 58 104 people were killed, 7876 injured, and 10 556 listed as missing in the city of Tokyo alone. In Tokyo prefecture, the number of deaths reached 59 593 and the number of missing 10 904. In Yokohama there were 265 000 casualties. Ito settlement, with a population of 14 000, disappeared into the ocean, leaving no trace behind. The report gives the following total estimated figures: 93 331 deaths, 43 476 missing, and 103 733 severely injured. About 3 300 000 people were left homeless [215].

The Japanese have learned from this tragedy. Now, in planning the construction of houses they take into consideration the possibility of such a catastrophe and its most damaging consequence, fire. Fire shelters have been built in Tokyo, providing protection for 70 000 in 30 min. A special Central Council, with local branches in Tokyo, Nogaya, and Osaka, has been established to work on effective measures for preventing such catastrophes. A standard method has been developed for determining the seismological stability of hospitals, schools, fire brigade buildings, and police stations. Special methods of combating fire and for the efficient evacuation of the population are also being thoroughly researched [47].

But people do not always learn from the lessons of the past. Blinkered and conservative people prefer to ignore them, and others will consciously risk a tragedy in order to gain other benefits. The earthquake on February 4, 1976 cost the Guatemalan people approximately 25 000 lives – 77 000 were injured and 258 000 buildings were destroyed. Almost a million remained homeless. As is clear from the Keno report (cited in [47]), the basic reason for such tragic consequences was the low seismic stability of the region and the low quality of construction in general.

It is impossible to determine the precise natural reason for a distaster, and of course we cannot prevent it.

Japanese seismologists register an annual average of 7500 earthquakes. Every 24 h in the USSR 10–15 earthquakes occur, i.e., roughly 3000–5000 annually. Of these, 100–200 are actually felt and may cause damage to buildings. Each year five earthquakes of a magnitude similar to (or even stronger than) that in Tashkent on April 26, 1966 occur. Including the Kuril-Kamchatka zone, the number of strong earthquakes reaches 20–25 a year. Two to three earthquakes of high magnitude take place annually in central Asia [219]. Periodically occurring earthquakes and sometimes subsequent tsunami are also registered in other seismoactive and tsunami-active zones of the world.

Data provided by the Secretary General of the International Union of Geodesics and Geophysics show that the average annual number of lives lost due to earthquakes reaches 15 000. In the ten-year period 1948–1957 more than a million people died as victims of earthquakes, volcanic eruptions, cyclones, and floods [215]. Together with periodically occurring famine and increasing traumatism (especially in the case of road traffic catastrophes), natural disasters account for a significant proportion of mortality and disease in the world.

As noted by Belousov et al. [37], the potential danger of earthquakes is growing – not because they are becoming stronger, but because in many countries situated in seismically active zones the construction of high buildings goes on, in spite of the warnings of seimologists. In addition, new causes of earthquakes, those of an anthropogenic character, have recently arisen. Growth and concentration of population in seismically active, tsunami-active, and mudflow zones and the industrial development in these areas will also increase the damage resulting from natural disasters.

For example, the capital of Kazakhstan, Alma-Ata (formerly Vernyi), was struck by devastating earthquakes (9–10 on the Richter scale) in 1887 and 1911, and by mudflows with catastrophic consequences in 1921 and 1963. Meanwhile, the city's population is constantly growing: from 45 600 in 1926 to 776 000 in 1972, a 17-fold increase.

San Francisco lies in a dangerous quake-prone zone. Nonetheless, in the region of the San Andreas Fault (a gigantic cleft 1000 km long) intensive construction continues. Annually, almost 50 new projects are launched in this area [276]. Buildings are erected even on steep mountain slopes and in the valleys of the fault, vulnerable to floods. It is a fatal mistake, and a misunderstanding of the significance of the danger, not to take these local circumstances into consideration by implementing special preventive measures.

In spite of the lessons of the past, the tendency remains to ignore the laws of nature and to maintain a blinkered attitude toward the loss of control over a population's health and safety. The present investigation analyzes selected, historically documented natural disasters, in order to illustrate the scope of the problem and its place in human development.

In most cases, the irreversible consequences of natural disasters, including those for public health, were predetermined by:

1. Absence of efficient protective constructions, resulting in enormous damage and many injuries, as in Hamburg after the flood of February 16–17, 1961 [111]
2. Disregard or underestimation of potential danger, as in Honolulu (1958, 1959), where – though warned twice – people did not believe there was a real threat and therefore did not move to safer ground [214]
3. Lack of the knowledge (regarding causes and warning signs) needed to organize preventive measures, as in the tsunami which damaged the Kuril Islands (USSR) on November 4–5, 1952 [32]

4. Ignorance, disregard, or misinterpretation of facts connected with natural disasters, leading to indifference and risk-taking rather than prevention, as in the past and at present in Algeria, Iran, Italy, Morocco, Turkey, etc.

An earthquake in Argentina on March 20, 1861 destroyed the towns of Mendou, San Juan, and Cordova, killing 18 000 people. On January 15, 1944 another strong quake destroyed San Juan, killing 5000 of its 80 000 inhabitants and injuring another 10 000. All the hospitals of the town were destroyed and the water supply system and electric cables no longer functioned. The entire population had to be evacuated immediately [248].

The implementation of preventive and protective measures is not only a question of huge material investments. What is frequently lacking in a situation of extreme emergency is preliminary planning for the mobilization of available means and forces, medical and sanitary included, at the focus of the disaster within a few hours of its occurrence. In earthquake-prone areas, three things are of primary importance: antiseismic construction, prognostication, and prevention of damage.

Much has been done by the Tokyo International Institute of Seismology and Seismically Stable Constructions. In the USSR an Interministerial Council of Seismology and Seismically Stable Constructions has been functioning under the organizational framework of the Academy of Science Presidium, which determined its activities as research and development. The Sakhalin Research and Development Institute and the Soviet Hydro-meteorological Service are responsible for forecasting tsunami; a special commission for research on mudflows, coordinated by the Academy of Sciences of the USSR, has also been established.

My own experience and research indicate that in the USSR and other countries the medical aspects of problems related to natural disasters are considerably underestimated. There is no comprehensive, systematic study of the problem in the available literature. Some research concerning public health under conditions created by natural disasters, including descriptions of the psychological state of the population, was published in Russia in the late nineteenth and early twentieth centuries [27, 142]. Bazhenov [27], observing the Azov flood (1914), noted the appearance of short-term psychoses and long-term nervous disturbances. The symptoms were related to traumatic hysteria or traumatic neurosis.

The low level of public health services in Russia at that time did not allow for provision of appropriate medical aid to the injured, on the one hand because of the extreme dispersion of responsibilities between various organizations, and on the other because of insufficient equipment. According to information provided by Marshansky in 1913, the extra-hospital network of health services in Russia consisted of 1230 dispensaries, and the number of beds in stationary hospitals was 49 087. In the whole of Russia, 24 000 physicians were registered [277].

This state of things, as well as the lack of coordination between the many branches of the health services, is typical for many countries, even today. Lack of means and material prevented these organizations from taking even the basic steps to deal with the public health consequences of natural disasters. In fact, such measures were never even considered!

We can judge the real capabilities of the health services in Russia at that time from such facts as the following: In 1914 the entire medical service of the Caspian region consisted of one medical division with one doctor and one medical assistant, and five additional dispensary stations with one medical assistant each [232]. An inquiry carried out by the Pirogov Society showed that 19 of 52 large urban centers had no public health physicians; only some of them (Baku, Yekaterinodar) had public health supervisors [278].

The First World War and the civil wars (1918–1921) and the famine that followed made the situation even worse. The health service system was destroyed; it is understandable that at this time attention was paid to issues other than natural disasters and their medical aspects.

The Crimean earthquake in 1927 received wide coverage in the USSR. Brusilovsky et al. [45] reported on its expectional force. Symson [231] and Podyapolsky [196] paid particular attention to its medical aspects. The problems of organization of medical aid to the injured and of dealing with the public health consequences of the earthquake remained untouched for a long time.

It was my duty to provide medical aid to the injured after the Tiraspol earthquake (November 9–10, 1940); a team on regular night duty at the emergency station and one ambulance were at my disposal. The quake happened suddenly, and the health service system was not prepared for rescue operations. The team on duty at the hospital to which the injured were evacuated, as well as those at other medical institutions, failed from the very beginning to provide appropriate management and coordination of the activities. Preliminary instructions for emergency cases did not exist; there was no possibility of receiving additional medical personnel, equipment, or other means of providing medical aid.

Reports on other natural disasters present the same picture [32]. The tragedy of the Ashkhabad earthquake provides a special lesson. The soviet writer Lazar Karelin [129] gives a picturesque but truthful précis of the event: "In Ashkhabad he did not see a single building standing. Only afterwards was he shown one house, the one built with seismically stable over-indulgence" (p. 251).

In May 1960 a signal warning of a possible tsunami was sent out in Kamchatka. The population was not ready for the calamity; no protective measures were undertaken, and no medical preparations were made. The bulk of the population, the medical personnel, and others knew nothing about the phenomenon, its possible effects, or its origin.

Extremely scanty and laconic information emerged from Daghestan after a catatrophic earthquake on May 14, 1970: "There was a landslide near Kalinin-aul. It came over the river, and the water reached the dwellings of the outlying region. There was danger of flood. Fresh wounds, fresh graves . . ." [279]. It is difficult to understand how medical aid was provided to the injured. Shafranskaya has written [220] that at the moment of danger people usually do not choose behavior most fitting to the situation.

It is obvious that when a natural disaster occurs, especially at its beginning, some delay in the deployment of rescue crews and other help is unavoidable. For this reason it is imperative that activities be organized within the general system of health services and environmental sanitation – before the disaster.

Throughout the world a great deal of experience and a vast amount of documentary materials have been accumulated concerning various natural disasters, classified by origin and resulting damages. Investigation of the medical aspects drawn from this material will provide the following:

1. An identification and classification of injuries and diseases following earthquakes, tsunami, floods, and other natural disasters
2. An acquaintance with approbated organizational systems of public protection, aid to the injured, and elimination of public health consequences of natural disasters
3. An analysis of mistakes made, elaboration of a rational system of prevention, and a corresponding system of efficient administration of aid to the injured under varying geographical conditions

In this respect the catastrophic earthquake in Guatemala in 1976 is instructive. First, it took place in a country where natural disasters are quite frequent, which means it was not regarded as an extraordinary phenomenon. It is thus to be expected that a well-established basis must exist there for efficient mobilization of resources to the site of a (predicted) calamity. At least the absence of such a basis seems irrational. During the period 1952–1976 alone, Guatemala suffered 20 large floods; four serious fires (including that of 1960, which happened in a neuropsychiatric hospital); six volcanic eruptions; five hurricanes and two tropical storms; two serious earthquakes (1958 and 1964); destruction of a dam (1958); and drought on the Atlantic coast (1975).

The 1976 earthquake happened at 3:33 on the morning of February 4. It struck one-third of the country, killing 24 340 and injuring 90 000. Meanwhile, 220 000 houses were destroyed and a million people were rendered homeless. Among the reasons for such heavy damage are the social aspects [15]. Such helplessness and inability in providing appropriate and efficient aid to the injured and clearing away the damage seems to occur with regularity. It was difficult to compensate for the lack of a previously established system of emergency activities and rescue operations. One event followed another as the situation became worse and worse. The steps taken in fact enabled only passive observation instead of efficient provision of aid.

A large number of landslides destroyed bridges and blocked the main route to the Atlantic, rivers, and lakes. Another quake struck the region at 12:20 on February 6, registering 5.75–6 on the Richter scale. The emotional effects of this disaster were especially acute, and the general state of shock greatly aggravated the situation. During the following 6 weeks thousands of earth movements were registered.

In this situation, coordination of efforts was imperative. However, nothing was done, according to a memorandum [230]. The Guatemalan Minister of Defense, designated head of the coordinating committee (which consisted of military officials), found himself isolated from other institutions and organizations. In particular, the committee contradicted the activities of the Guatemalan Ministry of Health. The Health Minister himself returned from abroad only 5 days after the earthquake. There was also no interaction between epidemiologists sent by the Central American Research Center and the Guatemalan coordinating committee.

Seriously lacking were reliable data on

a) the extent, character, and type of damages and injuries,
b) available means of aid in the stricken regions,
c) locations of those in need of medical aid and hospitalization, and
d) alternative mobile hospitals.

The numerous volunteers who came had no equipment, did not speak the local language, and had no idea of the local conditions and the kind of help needed. Frequently, the medicines, bandaging material, and vaccines which came from abroad were outdated or otherwise worthless.

In addition, the medical teams were not used efficiently. For example, an American preventive medicine team was assigned to the 47 US Field Hospital in Chimaltenango. As stated in the above-mentioned memorandum, this team could have been instrumental in evaluating the public health and safety conditions and could have been especially efficient in making the appropriate decisions. But it had no authority to expand its activities beyond the mentioned field hospital. Other obstacles to efficient work by the team were poor knowledge of the local language and lack of appropriate means of transportation.

The medical forces and others involved in providing aid after the quake were far from sufficient. Of four hospitals within the Guatemalan health care system, only two were functioning after the earthquake on February 4th. For the first 2 days these hospitals worked in isolation, using their own limited personnel without help from outside [15].

It became obvious that the Guatemalan Health Ministry was incapable of coordinating a national program for dealing with the aftermath of the quake. As expected, acute hygiene problems arose. There was a 40% reduction in the water supply in Guatemala City, and the water shortage was also felt in the agricultural regions. It was impossible to prevent pollution of the water by precipitation and feces. The endemic problem of malnutrition in Guatemala was aggravated, its main victims being the children. This was the price the country paid for being unprepared for an emergency situation.

The following groups must participate in a unified system, interconnected and interrelated with the nationwide health program, to provide organized medical aid:

1. The Ministry of Health
2. Various volunteer organizations
3. Social services
4. Private physicians

The most favourable circumstances were in the capital, Guatemala City, where 15% of the country's population lives. It is only natural that the main forces and means in any field, including the health service system, are concentrated in the capital. Yet this city is vulnerable to frequent natural disasters. It was totally destroyed by the earthquake in 1541, and then reconstructed. But again in 1874, and even more severely in 1917–1918, it suffered strong quakes. These are historical facts. It seems that the Guatemalan authorities have drawn conclusions from them, but have found it impossible to make and implement decisions. Helplessness and irrationalness are direct results of unresolved contradictions in the society, of both an inner and an outer nature. It is easy to acquire new technology, new armaments; however, Spinoza said that in their actions, people are led by superficial affect rather than by wisdom. And as most people are of a conservative mind, the way is even more difficult: *primum bonus* does not always occur in harmony with *summum bonus*.

Serious consideration of the natural disaster problems in Guatemala indicates that effective decisions cannot be made without curing the basic social and economic ills of the country. This is also characteristic of other countries, especially those predisposed to natural disasters, to which problem can be added the effects of specific local geographical, historical, and developmental features.

An instructive example here is Itály, one of the most densely populated countries in Europe. Its southern half is prone to frequent earthquakes of high magnitude (e.g., 1908, 1968, 1980).

Tsunami and floods have also been registered there. Most important have been the lessons learned from errors and misconceptions, and the effects of loss of control in the emergency situation following natural disasters. Human losses have been enormous, especially after the earthquake and subsequent tsunami at Messina in 1908. However, the measures undertaken after the catastrophes to prevent such high losses in the future have been inexcusably insufficient. The town of Fiumicino was damaged by a sea wave in 1959, and in 1964 Longarone was destroyed by a flood and a landslide. In panic, 37% of the population of Pozzuoli fled from the town in 2 days upon receiving information of volcanic activity at Vesuvius in 1970.

A tragic earthquake in Italy on November 23, 1980, the delayed reaction to it, and the inefficient rescue operations are further witness to the lack of preparedness there. The event was apprehended as a national disaster, and the Minister of Interior Affairs was obliged to resign. Data given to the press on November 27, 1980 included the following figures: 8000 injured, 2800 dead, 1300 missing, 200 000 homeless. The lack of preparedness was widely discussed.

In 1979, 1981, and 1982 I visited Italy and made the following observations:

1. Inadequate measures for dealing with the injurious effects of floods in Venice and tsunami in Messina
2. Seismic instability of residential buildings, particularly in old quarters (e.g., Naples)
3. Environmental pollution and lack of hygiene (Rome, Venice, Naples, Milan, etc.)
4. Inadequacy of the transportation system and public utilities

These facts are well known to the Italian people, their government and institution, including the Ministry of Health, but the majority of the urgent problems connected with natural disasters remain, because of unresolved social and economic issues in the country.

Guatemala and Italy are situated on different continents and have nothing in common with respect to history, social and economic development, culture, geography, etc. However, the attidudes towards dealing with natural disasters are identical in both countries.

Another significant aspect is the military. In a way, natural disasters can be compared to military operations, if we consider the extent of their injurious effects [27]. A natural disaster resembles modern war with nuclear weapons, which cause horrendous damage. The consequences of modern war can be compared only to those of earthquakes and storms [125]. The bombs dropped on Hiroshima and Nagasaki in 1945 (each equivalent to 20 000 tons of TNT) killed 106 000 and injured 97 000. According to the press, a million people were injured and hundreds of thousands died as a result of the earthquake in Tien Shan, China, on July 28, 1976. The fear that an age of gigantic calamities awaits mankind seems well grounded – whole cities and even entire countries can disappear from the face of the earth [264].

This brief historical review of some natural disasters and of the present situation as observed in specific cases enables us to distinguish two principal periods:

1. One of ignorance about the main causes and characteristics of natural disasters, together with a lack of personnel and means with which to combat them. This leads to passivity in planning and implementing a complex system of prevention and protection
2. One of development of science and technology applicable to natural disasters and prediction of them. This makes prevention and protection possible

Modern development has opened the way for active interference by man, who is now equipped with the appropriate tools to influence the public health and safety conditions of his environment and to solve the problems stemming from natural disasters.

Taking into consideration historical experience and practical expediency, it seems reasonable to differentiate natural disasters according to their main causes:

1. Disasters of natural origin(seismic, meteorological, hydrological, volcanic etc)
2. Disasters of an anthropogenic character (those caused by man's activities)

Disasters in the first group cannot be prevented, but as far as those in the second group are concerned, it is man's duty to ensure sanitation of the environment, planning and supervision of the location of residential areas, and the development of hydrological, industrial, and other plants as well as public health services for the population.

It is also important to enforce control of some activities, such as transportation and traffic regulation, and to deal efficiently with automobile accidents and the injuries resulting from them. Among disasters of anthropogenic origin we must emphasize the devastating fires started by people in states of pathological depression. From reports in the press in February 1983, fires (due to drought and high winds) in Australia raged over an area of more than 200 000 km^2, killing 71 people and leaving 10 000 homeless. It is a well-grounded assumption that in at least one case in five the cause of fire was arson. Special data from the US national commission on problems of fire prevention show that in 2.5 million fires in the United States in 1972 there were 300 000 casualties, 12 000 of them fatal.

In many cases combined calamities are registered (earthquakes with tsunami, earthquakes with floods), and sometimes they are accompanied by famine. The following factors determine the gravity of the consequences of natural disasters and the way in which they must be handled:

1. Extent of territory damage; significant features of the territory and its population, e.g., hydrological, industrial, and other constructions, transportation systems
2. Magnitude and duration of the disaster and its effects, as well as the combined effects of simultaneous disasters
3. The socioeconomic situation of the country

4. Geographical peculiarities and the ethnic structure, composition and character of the population
5. The state of the public health services

The following chapters consider these factors and detail a system of measures to be undertaken in dealing with the public health consequences of various kinds of natural disasters.

Public Health Consequences of Earthquakes

Earthquakes are closely connected with all aspects of geological time [97], and the history of tectonic movements deforming the earth's crust provides us with important information on the earth's structure. In seismically active zones, earthquakes, as dynamic sequences of the system of deep cracks in the earth, are an unavoidable phenomenon, predetermined by natural laws.

The damaging effects of earthquakes are a serious problem for man. They vary in extent and character because of

a) topographical changes caused by landslides, damming of rivers, breaks in mountain reservoirs, etc.;
b) the impact of destroyed constructions (see Figs. 1–4 [189]); and
c) fires and other factors.

Earthquakes violate the regular conditions of the environment and the stability of the way of life. People are killed. Morbidity and mortality soar. Certain characteristics are typical for seismically active zones during and after strong earthquakes.

There are 100 000 earthquakes annually on our planet, most of them occurring in the Pacific Ocean [23]. South of the Philippine Islands, the Mediterranean seismic zone joins the Pacific zone; 15% of all earthquakes occur in this area.

The long-term seismic activity for a given area can be determined by noting the frequency and intensity of seismic shocks there over a given period of time. According to Riznichenko [212], the frequency of seismic shocks must be the main index of the degree of seismic danger for an area. A similar average for points over large territories is the geophysical basis for defining seismic regions.

Precise localization of earthquakes according to their intensity is the subject of regional and microseismic mapping, which requires knowledge of geomorphological, hydrogeological, and engineering conditions. Data from regional and microseismic maps are used in planning construction and civil engineering activities in seismically active zones. For example, in planning for the construction of important buildings such as hospitals it is imperative to consider the characteristics of the soil, e.g., oscillation and geolocical shifting [150].

Not only the effects of earthquakes, but also the frequency of their occurrence in a given area must be considered, and it is important to evaluate their potential force [219]. Table 1 summarizes the frequency of strong, catastrophic earthquakes in the USSR between 1868 and 1968 [32, 35].

As can be seen from the table, an average of two or more earthquakes occur within one generation in these seismically active zones. Some of these regions are

Table 1. Frequency of strong earthquakes in the USSR, 1868–1968

Seismic zone	No. of earthquakes 1868–1918	1918–1968	Frequency (years)
Precarpathians	3	1	4–36
Crimea	2	2	1–54
Caucasus	2	8	2–12
Kopet-Dag	1	3	2–34
Other regions of Central Asia	9	6	2–17
Altai	1	1	36
Transbaikalia	1	2	7–72
Far East	–	6	4–29
Total	19	29	

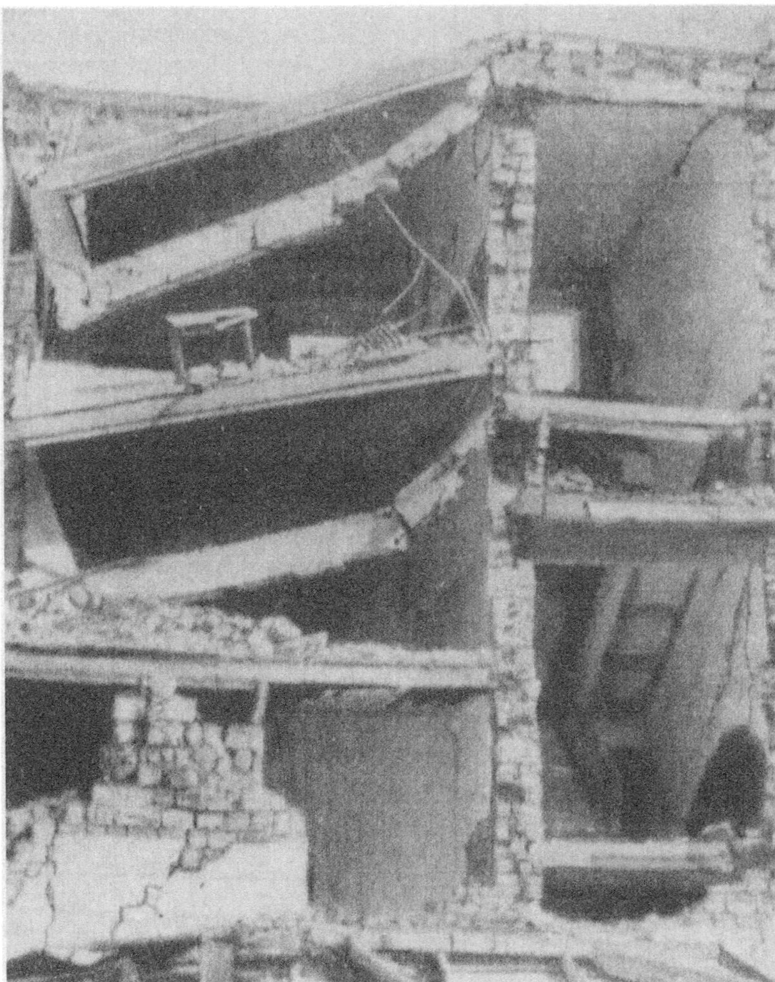

Fig. 1a, b. Railway School, city of Ashkhabad, after the earthquake in 1948. **a** The full-height collapse of the wall of the southwest past of the building. **b** see p. 14

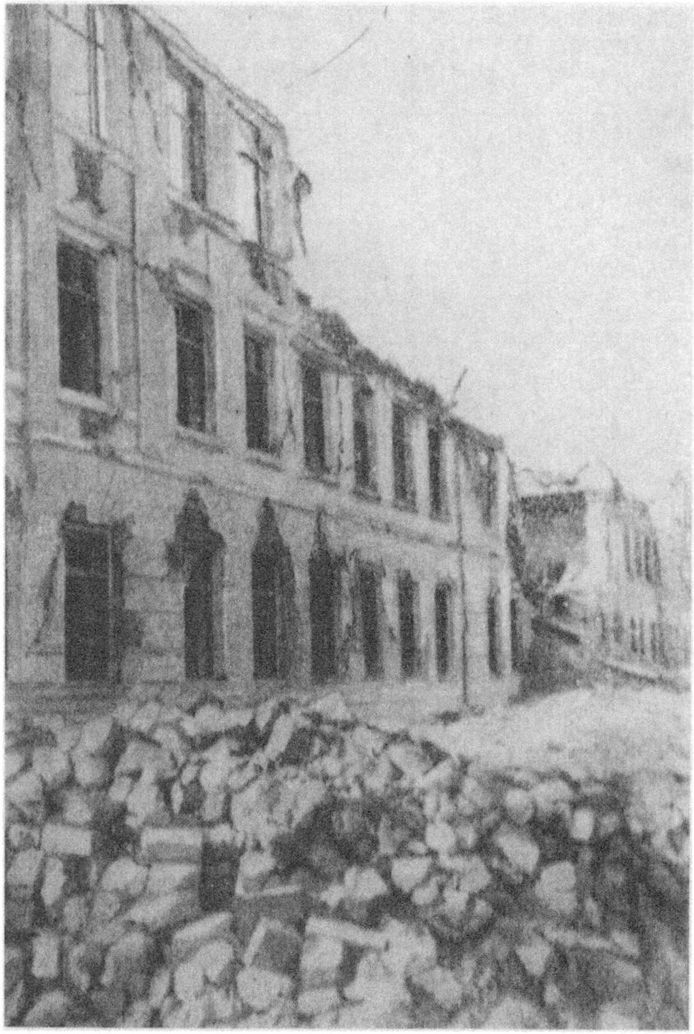

Fig. 1. **b** Main facade [189]

vulnerable as well to accompanying tsunami, floods, mudflows, or snowslides. Thus, in certain territories, the inherent physicogeographical conditions constitute a powerfully adverse influence on the environment and the health of the population [21]. In summarizing the past, Table 1 also becomes a prognostication.

The effect of earth tremors on volcanos, mountains, rivers, and lakes adds to the danger. These accompanying phenomena are also characteristic for certain areas. The Daghestan earthquake of May 14, 1970 and subsequent earth tremors brought about avalanches and landslides, damming the Sulak river and causing additional destruction and injuries. A day before the 1976 quake in Guatemala, the Panai

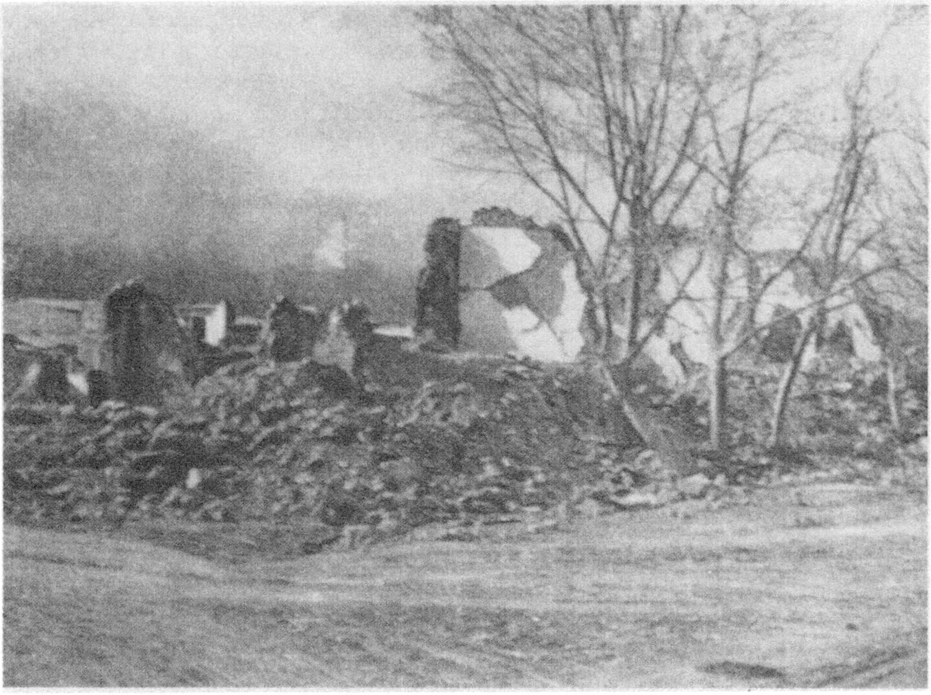

Fig. 2. Clay houses destroyed in the settlement of Geok-Tepe [189]

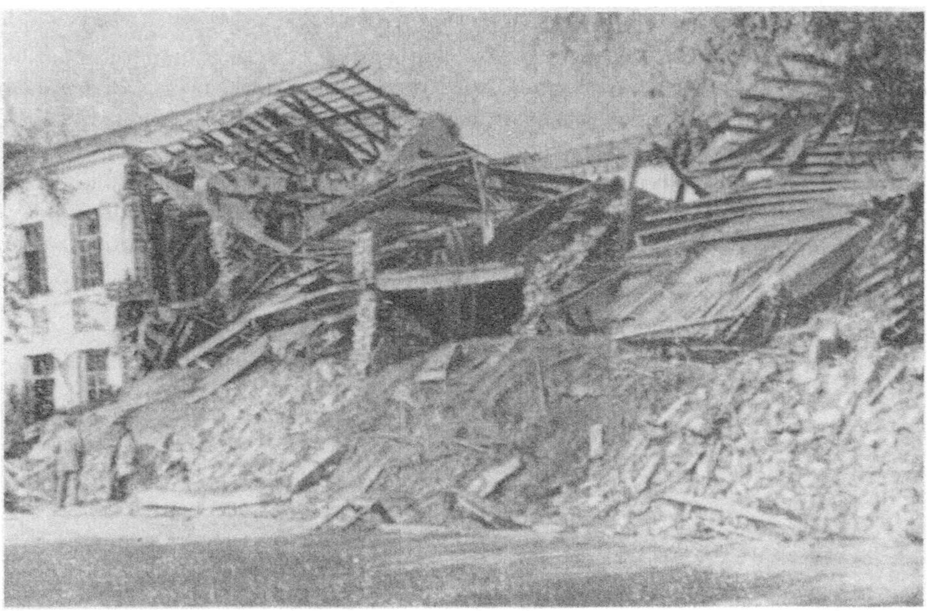

Fig. 3. Demolished center of the building housing the Academy of Science, Turkmen Soviet Socialist Republic [189]

volcano erupted, triggering large landslides which dammed the rivers near the towns of Patsua and San Martín; two lakes were formed. The devastation covered an area of 9065 km^2.

The countries most frequently struck by strong earthquakes are Algeria, Greece, Iran, Italy, China, the Latin American nations, Rumania, the Soviet Union, the United States, Turkey, Yugoslavia, and Japan. These countries lie in highly active seismic zones. Alone in Tadzhikistan, USSR, there have been 20 earthquakes of a magnitude greater than 8 on the Richter scale since 1895. Three were catastrophic in terms of damage to lives and property. The Karatagsky quake (1907) on the southern spurs of the Gissarsky range registered a magnitude of 8–10; 1000 people were killed and 150 villages were destroyed. The Sarezmian or Pamirian quake (1911) was followed by a huge landslide which destroyed the village of Usoi; the village of Sarez was the victim of the flooding of the Murgab River, dammed by the Landslide, which was 600–700 m high and 4 km wide, extending for 6 km. The Khaitsky quake (1949) caused a landslide from the top of Chokurak Mountain into the canyon of the Obi-Dara-Khauz River, totally burying the administrative center of the region, Khait, and devastating an area of 600 km^2 [144].

Many areas regarded as seismically active are densely populated. Here, Georgia must be mentioned; during the period 1920–1970 it was struck by nine devastating quakes; Gori (1920), Tabatzkur (1940), Gudamakar (1947), Gorno-Tushet (1951), Kakhetinian (1953), Gegechkor (1957), Achigvar (1960), Chkhaltinian (1963), and Borzhomi (1970) [182].

A similar situation is observed in the Carpathian-Balkan region, the seismically most dangerous zone in Europe, where there have been three catastrophic earthquakes since 1940. Seismic events are particularly frequent and intensive on the Adriatic coast, i.e., Yugoslavia, Albania, Bulgaria, Greece, and western Turkey [132].

In zones of extreme seismic activity, and against a background of intensive industrial development, constant population growth takes place. Fig. 4 and 5 show a huge increase in population density in recent decades, concentrated in large cities. Obviously, such growth aggravates the incidence and consequences of earthquakes. In some of these regions, gigantic artifical water reservoirs are responsible for an increase in the frequency of earthquakes. Researchers at the Athens Seismological Institute report a connection between a reservoir and subterranean tremors which

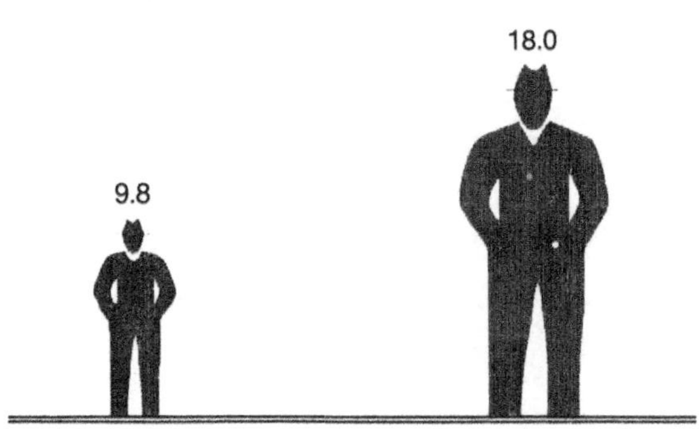

Fig. 4. Population density in Tadzik Soviet Socialist Republic (people/km^2)

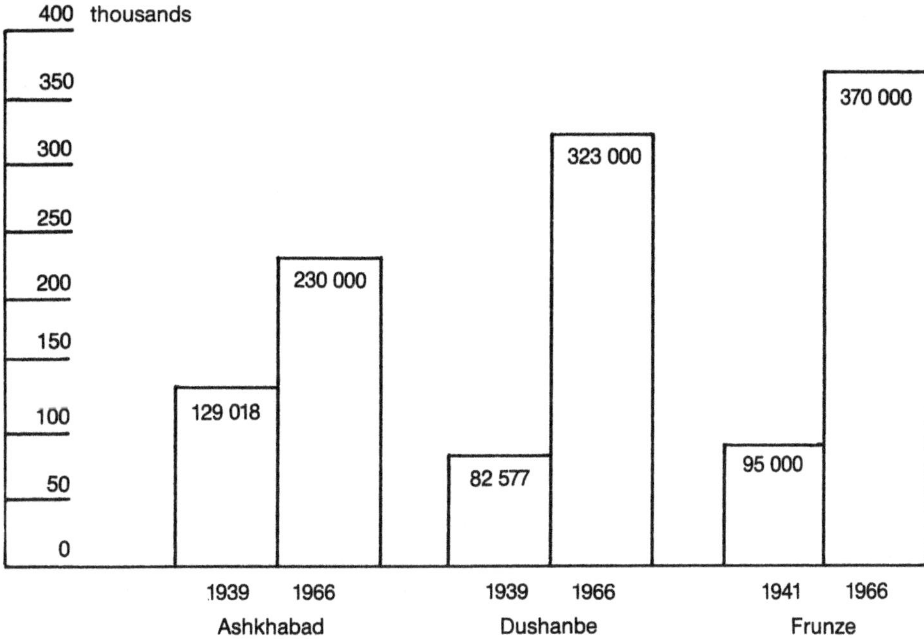

Fig. 5. Population growth in the cities of Ashkhabad, Dushanbe, and Frunze

destroyed 41 settlements in Euritania (Greece) in January 1966. Investigations showed that water in the storage lake exerted a pressure reaching 150 tons/m^2 on the underlying bedrock. The pressure caused shifting of huge geological formations, sharply increasing the seismic activity of the region. Lane [148] wrote that the occurrence of "dam earthquakes" is influenced by: the high density of the ground; additional artifical density created by the weight of water in reservoirs; water saturation of the skeleton pores in the rock and changes in ground water levels; existing cracks in the bedrock and delay in the transference of fluid pressure changes; and the effect of water as a lubricant, with consequent decrease in the friction of closed cracks and detachments.

Thus appear earthquakes of an anthropogenic character, their causes interconnected with natural ones. Modern technology and scientific progress make it possible to some extent to prevent the injurious effects of earthquakes. For example, a seismically stable, 36-story building has been constructed in the center of Tokyo. Unfortunately, such planning is not typical for most vulnerable areas, and preventive measures are far from satisfactory. Fatalities due to earthquakes remain intolerably high, as shown in Table 2 [32].

Often, these injuries are the direct or indirect consequences of

a) inadequate methods of construction and prevention,
b) population density, and
c) unsatifactory organization of rescue operations and medical aid.

Table 2. Earthquakes fatalities

Location	Date	Fatalities	Comment
Portugal [118]	1755	60 000	
China [175]	1850	Hundreds of thousands	
Italy [196]	1908	77 283	45.9% of population of Messina
USSR (Ashkhabad)	1948	23 282 [280, p. 125]	Unofficial sources reported 33 000 killed
Chile [214]	1960	10 000	
Turkey [281]	1966	2 394	
Iran [282]	1968	20 000	
Guatemala [47]	1976	25 000	

This situation could be improved through applied analysis of earthquakes, as outlined in Table 3.

There are concrete actions which should be taken to combat the effects of an earthquake, especially the irreversible human losses and the spread of general and infectious disease. The proportion of lost or severely injured may reach from 16% to 50% of the total population of a stricken area (San Juan, Argentina, 1944; Agadir, Morocco, 1960). This proportion determines the scope and character of medical aid provided. It must be noted here that there is usually a discrepancy between the needs and the possibilities where medical aid in emergencies is concerned.

Among the injured, women and children prevail. During the Ashkhabad earthquake, 47% of those killed were women, 35% children, and 18% men. The same

Table 3. Origin, consequences, and reasons for increased threat of earthquakes (in seismically active regions)

Origin
Seismic (unavoidable)
Anthropogenic (connected with man's activity)
Consequences
Deaths and injuries
Destruction of residential and other buildings
Secondary phenomena (tsunami, floods, fires etc.)
Sociological and environmental changes
Reasons for increased threat
Increased population density
Intensive industrialization, construction of hydroelectric buildings
Unsolved ecological problems
Prevention of injuries, protection, and aid
Implementation of antiseismic measures on the basis of:
a) regional and microseismic definition of seismic regions,
b) taking into consideration the geographic peculiarities of seismoactive zones
Elaboration and provision of a flexible system of measures including:
a) help to the injured, including medical aid,
b) elimination of the consequences, including the public health

ratio was reported in the Tashkent earthquake of April 1966, where five of the seven people killed in the first shock on the 26th were women; there were 1.5 times as many women wounded as men. According to Soviet sources (Freidlin), men are generally much more vulnerable to traumatic injuries than are women, statictics showing a ratio of 2:1. The reason why more women than men tend to be injured and killed in earthquakes is that a higher proportion of women are at home, indoors, and are therefore more vulnerable when buildings are damaged or completely destroyed. In addition to the seismic instability of residential constructions, women and children are naturally less mobile than men and less decisive in their actions when it comes to self-preservation. They are also subject to greater emotional stress in the face of an emergency, often resulting in a morbid helplessness.

The severe consequences of earthquakes are felt much more in urban than in rural areas. In Ashkhabad itself, those killed in the 1948 quake comprised 13.95% of the city's population, while in the nearby rural region of Geok-Tepenski the losses were 11.3% [280, pp. 59–113]. Specifically urban difficulties include rescuing the injured from under the ruins of high buildings; greater frequency of fires and explosions; more time needed to administer first aid and to evacuate the population in general and those needing hospitalization in particular. Trauma of epidemic proportions commonly follows a catastrophic earthquake. There is a constant ratio of killed to injured, with a large part of the latter severely injured. A substantial proportion of the population becomes homeless and must be evacuated. A general idea of the correlation between killed and injured in earthquakes can be grasped from Table 4 [32], which shows a ratio of killed to injured ranging from 1:0.34 to 1:15.3. From Table 4 we can also draw some conclusions as to the effectiveness of the emergency measures taken and the medical help provided, especially in the period directly following the calamity.

Figure 6, compiled on the basis of reports of the Ashkhabad [280, pp. 59, 113] and Tashkent [287] earthquakes, completes the general description of the injured. The Ashkhabad data emphasize the high index of irreversible losses (28.6%) and the high proportion (9.6%) of servere/medium traumas. According to Vishnevsky [280], 60% of the dead had injuries to the skull, spinal column, pelvis, or thorax. These injuries can be attributed to the character and magnitude of the quake, and to the

Table 4. Ratio of killed to injured at earthquakes

Date and place	Killed	Injured			Ratio of killed to injured	Comment
		Severely	Slightly	Total		
1929, North Iran [2]	3 253	NR	NR	1 121	1:0.34	
1930, Tadzhikistan [283]	151	61	147	208	1:1.4	
1931, Armenia [284]	231	324	558	882	1:3.8	
1934, Armenia [285]	456	NR	NR	1 189	1:2.6	
1943, Java [37]	213	1 165	2 096	3 261	1:15.3	58.1% of those severely injured died
1960, Morocco [286]	12 000	NR	NR	12 000	1:1	
1963, Yugoslavia [286]	2 000	883	2 500	3 383	1:1.7	
1976, Guatemala [270]	22 000	74 000	NR	NR	1:3.4	

NR, not reported

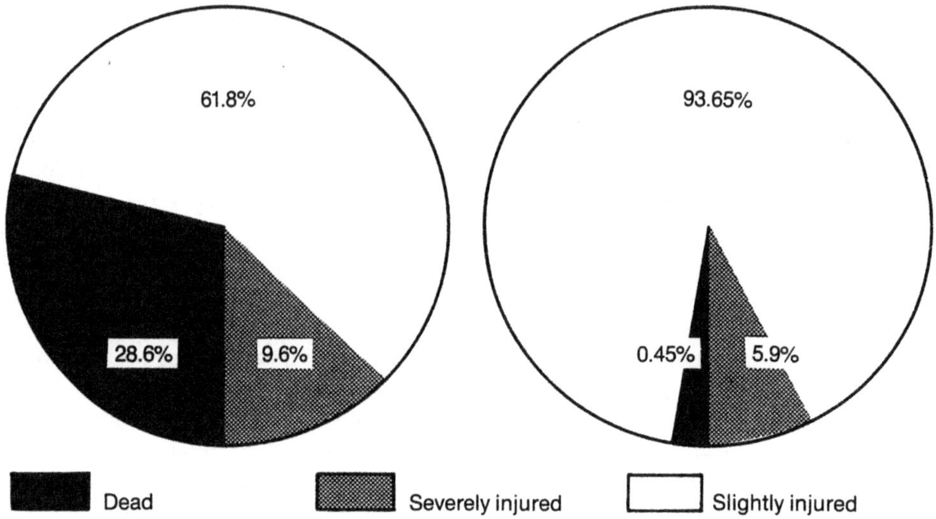

Fig. 6a, b. Earthquake casualties. **a** Ashkhabad, 1948. **b** Tashkent, 1966 (from a survey conducted April 30, 1966)

incompetence of the authorities responsible for prevention, rescue operations, and provision of medical aid. The Tashkent quake killed a relatively small proportion of the population (0.45%). Many more were injured. Large numbers of people became ill, especially from infectious diseases. Many were left homeless; 84 000 apartments, 225 children's institutions, and 181 schools were destroyed [254].

Earthquakes frequently cause fires, which also bring about widespread damage. Of 150 000 people killed in the Japanese quake of September 1, 1923, two-thirds were the victims of fires [248]. As a result of the quake on the Greek island of Ithaki during the night of August 10–11, 1953, the town of Zakinph was totally destroyed by fire [137].

As we see, the appearance of fires after earthquakes resembles conditions of war in which atomic weapons are used. After the explosion of the atomic bombs in Hiroshima and Nagasaki in 1945, 100 000 people suffered from burns. Of note here is the impact of the victims' behavior with regard to their own rescue and self-preservation. In Tashkent, 55% of the traumatic injuries were the result of inappropriate behavior – jumping from upper floors of buildings, colliding with objects in the panic of escape [12].

The magnitude an character of the earthquake, the extreme geographical conditions, and the safety and rescue measures undertaken may alter the figures on damages. Yet the general picture remains more or less typical, even though there are data reliable enough to make prediction possible and to plan for an emergency situation. The high percentage of deaths and severe injuries shown in Fig. 6 for the Ashkhabad quake is evidence of the inability of local forces to effectively cope with such an emergency. Emergency bases must be created in regions near those known

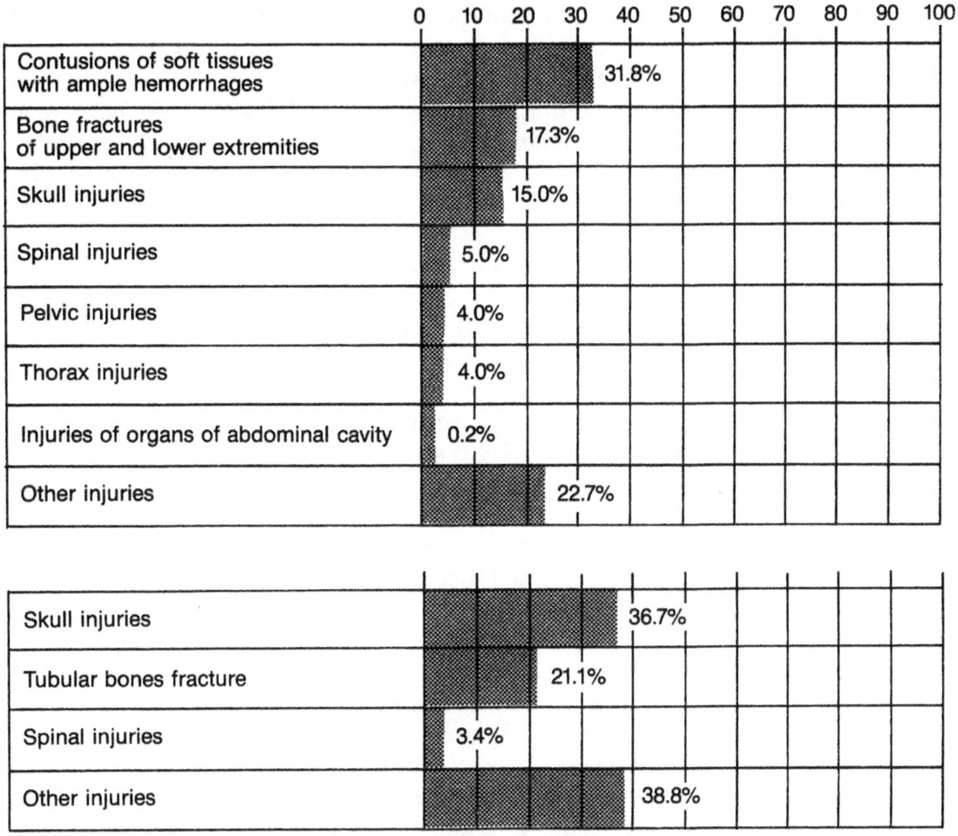

Fig. 7. Types of injuries requiring hospitalization of casualties after the earthquakes at Ashkhabad, 1948 **(above)** and Tashkent, 1966 **(below)**

to be vulnerable to natural disasters. To this end the possible problems and types of damage to be encountered must be considered. Fig. 7 is elaborated from data on the Ashkhabad quake [280, pp. 109–110] (specifiying 4000 cases) and the Tashkent quake [287]. The majority of those evacuated to hospitals suffered injuries to soft tissue (contusions, lacerations, etc.). In Ashkhabad these comprised 31.8% of the injured. According to Petrova and Kamilov [195], who reported from the Tashkent earthquake, soft tissue injuries there accounted for 72.5% of all injuries, i.e., 2.2 times more than at Ashkhabad. Skull traumas followed soft tissue injuries in proportion, reaching 36.7% at Tashkent. This is almost 2.5 times more than the corresponding proportion at Ashkhabad (15%). In accounting for the percentage differences between the two kinds of injuries at the two sites, the main reason appears to have been the delayed and ineffective provision of aid in Ashkhabad in 1948. Obviously, there was a high mortality of injured at the site of the disaster, while mortality was lower among those evacuated and/or hospitalized.

The recovery of those with skull traumas is very dependent on quick provision of medical aid. This is vividly illustrated by data from the Second World War, between the Soviet Union and Germany, 1941–1945. About half (47%) of those who had closed trauma to the skull died during the first 24 h. In 14.5% of cases death came within 2 h after injury. Thus, almost half of the injured died before reaching specialized hospitals and, therefore, without having received any qualified aid [101]. After the Ashkhabad earthquake the situation was similar. The proportion of tubular bone fractures was 3.8% higher in the Tashkent earthquake than at Ashkhabad. This appears to be so because of the higher mortality of those so injured at Ashkhabad. Unfavorable conditions there also resulted in a higher mortality for those with traumas of the spine, pelvis, and thorax.

Military experience shows that multiple fractures of the spinal column are incurred when collapsing constructions fall on people who are standing. Severe injuries of the spinal column and the spinal cord are also met when stone or wooden constructions fall on people who are lying down [100].

The "crush syndrome" is one of the serious effects of earthquakes. Kuzin [146] noted this in 3.5% of the injured at Ashkhabad, though this figure appears low. According to Krols, Miroi, and Yugono (cited in Shamov et al. [221]), crush syndrome with renal insufficiency was observed in 69 of 87 injured. Seven of 19 persons with tubular bone fractures were classified as cases of prolonged crush syndrome [287].

The striking difference between crush syndrome data registered in Ashkhabad and reports provided from other catastrophes can be explained by the fact that in Ashkhabad a large proportion of the victims of this syndrome died at the site of injury, before medical aid arrived.

The Tashkent earthquake of 1966 serves as an example of prolonged (up to a year) injurious effects of recurring underground tremors. Table 5, based on reports from the Tashkent first aid office, shows the distribution of disorders suffered by victims for the days of strong shocks.

It is very important to assess the character of injuries by location, especially in the immediate aftermath of a disaster, to determine what specialized medical aid is needed and to what extent evacuation is necessary. Table 6 characterizes the injuries sustained in the Ashkhabad quake by location [280, pp. 109–111]. Patients with minor wounds who applied for ambulatory surgical aid mostly had multiple injuries, according to the report of the Alma-Ata medical group functioning in Ashkhabad. Wounds of the extremities were prevalent (60%), and in 17% of cases the skull was injured [280, p. 92]. The number of patients (excluding traumatopathic cases) applying for medical aid at the beginning of the quake was relatively small. Among

Table 5. Victims of Tashkent earthquake, 1966 (Tashkent First Aid Office)

	Proportions of cases (%)	Proportions of hospital admissions (%)
Traumas	33.7	68.0
Cardiovascular diseases	23.6	3.3
Psychoneuroses	16.5	1.2

Table 6. Location of injuries incurred by victims of Ashkhabad earthquake, 1948

	Proportions of total (%)
Fractures of extremities and shoulder girdle	
Lower leg, foot	45
Shoulder, forearm	24
Thigh	22
Clavicle and shoulder blade	9
Head injuries	
Contusions	50
Scalp	11
Brain	11
Eye	9
Facial soft tissue	7
Nose and ear	5
Jaw	4
Fornix and base of skull	3
Injuries to thorax	
Rib fractures	56
Soft tissue injuries	40
Lung injuries	1.5
Subcutaneous emphysema	1.5
Hemothorax	1

the 4111 severely injured who were evacuated from the Ashkhabad military hospital, the diseased comprised 5% [280, p. 109].

The neuroemotional stress at the beginning of a disaster greatly affects the rate of neuropsychological and cardiovascular diseases. Shock psychosis is one frequently reported consequence of earthquakes. Dulling of the mind follows. Sometimes the stupor is preceded by motor excitement and senseless escape activity, as observed in both Ashkhabad and Tashkent. The psychosis continues for several hours. Residual phenomena in the form of attacks of fright may occur for a long time afterwards. After the Crimean earthquake, cases of increased vibrational sensitivity, sleep disturbances, deep syncopes, and stupors were noted [45].

After the Tiraspol earthquake in 1940 I observed victims suffering psychological misadaptation and reactive states. These cases came second in number to traumatic injuries. The proportion of people suffering from psychological disturbances after the Ashkhabad quake was especially significant. Of the patients delivered to the Republican psychiatric center of the Uzbek SSR Ministry of Health in 1948, 25% were victims of the earthquake. Among the 635 treated in Turkmenia by psychiatrists, the largest portion comprised cases of psychosis, neurosis, and psychoneurosis listed as complications of traumas received in the earthquake [288, pp. 13, 63]. Psychiatric patients comprised the same proportion of cases from the Tashkent earthquake [6]. On the days when there were strong underground tremors, 16.5% of those treated by the emergency medical services presented with psychoneurotic disorders [127].

Table 7. Incidence of myocardial infarction in three residential areas ot the city of Tashkent per 1000 of population aged >40

District	1964	1965	1966	1967	1968
Oktiabrsky	0.52	0.66	0.96	1.08	0.6
Kuibyshevsky	5.4	5.0	6.1	6.7	7.4
Chilanzarsky	0.69	0.97	1.33	1.77	1.58

Asthenia of the nervous system, combined with vegetative-vascular deviation, was observed in Tashkent both during strong tremors and a few month later. The aggravating situation caused complications in those suffering from cardiovascular diseases. There was an increase of 20.5% in cases related to cardiovascular pathology in 1966 compared with the previous year, and another increase of 27% in 1967 [127]; cases of myocardial infarction became especially frequent. During the period of the strongest tremors (April–December 1966) in Tashkent, these cases were twice as high in number as their average during the period 1961–1965 [253].

The number of patients treated for myocardial infarction in Tashkent clinical hospital No. 15 increased 3 and 2.5 times in 1966 respectively, compared with 1964 and 1965. The ratio of male to female patients was 2.35:1. Men were more exposed to prolonged emotional and physical stress and to unfavorable environmental conditions. Of those treated, 55.9% were aged 41–60, and 40% were over 60 [3].

The increase in cardiovascular cases was largely registered among the population coming from the residential areas near the epicenter of the earthquake. Table 7 demonstrates the proportions of myocardial infarction cases observed in the various regions of Tashkent [25]. During the period 1966–1967 all regions showed an increase in cases. This is directly related to the frequent underground tremors; more than 800 were recorded in the year following the earthquake. In the center of the city the intensity of the quake registered 8 on the Richter scale, in the outskirts, only 6 [254]. The Kuibyshevsky District was the epicenter of the quake. Correspondingly, the increase in myocardial infarctions there, was especially marked. The Oktiabrsky district was least susceptible in this respect; its population is comprised of Uzbeks, among whom the rate of myocardial infarctions is low. Figures pertaining to the Chilanzarsky district (which was least affected) were unfavorably influenced by the fact that it absorbed victims of other districts damaged by the earthquake. Earthquakes also cause increased complications for myocardial infarction patients; in Tashkent, mortality among such patients increased from 29.3% in 1965 to 34.8% in 1966 [253].

It is known that hypertension can have a psychogenic component. An earthquake not only promotes the possibiliy of hypertensive disorders, but also aggravates them. In Tashkent the number of such patients increased in 1966 by 18% and in 1967 by 48% [127].

Persons with high systolic blood pressure display surplus reactivity when under emotional and humoral stress. Of 2526 patients with cardiocerebral disease, 239 (9.4%) suffered complications caused by hypertensive crises. Men were twice as susceptible as women to such crises after the earthquake; the increase reported for the latter group was 13% [53]. Men normally suffer more than women from the aggravated course of hypertension, and the earthquake caused even more psychic and physical surplus tension in them.

Hypertensive crises complicated by coronary insufficiency became more frequent in connection with recurring underground tremors registering 7 on the Richter scale, between April 26 and 30 and between May 8 and 12, 1966 [195]. The first 2 months after the quake showed a considerable increase in hemorrhagic insults, from 10.1% in the corresponding period of the previous year to 16.8% in 1966.

Cerebral circulation disturbances in young people became frequent as well. In 1965 Those aged 30–50 comprised only 7.1% of such cases; after the earthquake in April 1966 this figure reached 12%. In older people (aged 50–60) the corresponding index of cerebral circulation disturbances showed an increase of 3% [156]. The reason for the increase detailed above were the psychoemotional effects of the quake on the victims, a change for the worse in their everyday living conditions, and the recurring underground tremors (up to 500 following the earthquake) [3, 156].

It became apparent that organization for prevention and protection was poor, and that treatment of the cerebral insult cases was unsatisfactory. Gradually, people calmed down, and the irritability caused by the underground tremors became more bearable; the psychoemotional reactions gradually diminished, then faded away. On October 13, 1966, although Tashkent was struck by a magnitude-7 tremor, no essential increase in hypertensive crises was reported. There had been a natural adaptation by the population to the new living conditions, and by then measures had been taken to diminish the injurious effects of the underground tremors.

Earthquakes also promote the appearance and aggravate the course of endocrine diseases. The Tashkent earthquake was followed by many cases of acute early and aggravated diabetes mellitus; blood sugar levels reached 500 mg and more, and glucosuria was reported at a level of 7%. There were frequent cases of diabetic coma, because worsened medical conditions prevented patients from receiving insulin; general stress and traumatic injuries were also contributing factors. Precomatose and comatose states may appear during the first few hours after the earthquake.

In May–June of 1966 Tashkent endocrinologists reported a worsening in 35 of 37 thyrotoxicosis cases and relapses in 50 of 55. During these 2 months the population was particularly susceptible to psychological tension because of strong (up to 7 on the Richter scale) recurring underground tremors [130].

Earthquakes also influence the course of pregnancies. Toxicosis in late pregnancy was registered in 8.3% of cases in Tashkent. Nephropathy also increased [204]. A quake unfavorably affects pregnant women and children, i.e., that part of the population least resistant to environmmental crisis. These consequences are illustrated by data provided by the health services of the Turkmen SSR [289, p. 80] on the mortality of mothers and children in Ashkhabad, compared with other cities and towns of the Turkmen Republic [32, 35]. Table 8 indicates that, compared with Krasnovodsk, Mary, and other regions, the mortality of mothers, prematurely born infants, and children in general, as well as the number of stillbirths, was much higher in Ashkhabad. The main reason was worsened conditions during the course of pregnancy and delivery. In Ashkhabad on October 14, 1948, 15 of 25 pregnant women gave birth normally, while in ten cases the birth either was premature or miscarried [280, p. 113].

Table 8. Postpartum and postnatal mortality, Turkmen SSR, 1949 (%)

Institution	Mothers	Full-term infants	Premature infants	Stillbirths
Turkmen Medical Institute, obstetrics and gynecology clinic	0.3	3.0	34.0	3.8
Krasnovodsk, maternity home	0.1	2.1	31.0	ND
Town of Mary, maternity home	0.07	2.3	18.0	ND
Mary region, maternity homes	ND	ND	ND	2.7
Chardzhousky, maternity home	ND	ND	ND	1.9

ND, no data

Disturbances in nutrition caused by lack of mothers' milk and overcrowding in children's homes were the main reasons for the high rate of dystrophy. In the Maryisky House for Children, hypotrophy comprised 75% of cases; in the Tashauzsky House, 65%; and in the Chardjousky House, 77%. This, in turn, influenced the children's physical development and predetermined the high child mortality, which in 1949 reached 25.7% in the Maryisky House, and 14.8% in the Chardjousky House. The children died of dysentery and other intestinal diseases (48%) and pneumonia (25%) [289, pp. 90, 91].

After a certain period of time following an earthquake, the unfavorable environmental conditions and people's reduced resistance result in an increase in the spread of infectious diseases. In the Turkmen SSR a year after the 1948 earthquake, there were twice as many cases of malaria as in the year of the quake itself. This was the result of

a) water pollution after the irrigation and water supply systems were destroyed, and
b) mass migration of the population, which facilitated the entry and spread of the malaria agent into the region.

The combined effects of epidemiological problems and inadequate medical aid brought about a sharp increase in acute intestinal infections and infectious diseases in children. In 1949 as compared with the previous year in Ashkhabad there were increases of 36% in typhoid, 32% in dysentery, 30% in diphtheria, and 15% in scarlet fever cases [290, pp. 94–96]. The index of measles cases (19 children per 1000) which were under treatment in 1948 increased to 27.3 in 1949, and the corresponding mortality increased from 4% to 5.2%.

Madzhidov [155] noted that a real threat of epidemics arose in Tashkent after the earthquake, especially of infectious intestinal deseases. In the summer and fall of 1966, 15%–16% of patients delivered to hospitals by ambulance suffered from acute intestinal diseases. Furthermore, the unsatisfactory living conditions, increased contact between children, and reduction of their immunobiological protective systems caused an epidemic of whooping cough [128]. Most of the victims were year-old children (5.6–8.5 per 1000), who could not be completely inoculated.

The Ashkhabad earthquake caused the spread of transmissible tropical diseases [90, 191]. The destroyed city became a breeding ground for mosquitoes – transmitters of dermal leishmaniasis. Their number increased drastically, and an epidemic of this disease (the urban type) struck the population in 1949–1950. A considerable

Table 9. Mortality by department in various medical treatment facilities, Turkmen SSR, 1947–1948 (%)

Department	1947	1948	Increase (%)
General medicine	2.1	3.0	40
Surgery	2.5	3.2	30
Pediatrics (tuberculosis)	4.3	14.3	230
Pediatrics (ear, nose, throat)	0.3	0.9	200
Infectious diseases (adults)	3.5	4.9	40
Psychiatry	0.1	1.8	1700

decrease in their number – from 216.4 on a sticksheet (lappula) in 1950 to 14.5 in 1953 – as a result of a program of insect and dog extermination brought about a drastic decrease in morbidity [191].

Injuries, unfavorable living conditions, and decreased resistance in the population following an earthquake all worsen the course of disease, with a resultant high mortality.

Table 9 compares the mortality after the 1948 earthquake with that of the previous year [291, p. 223]. As can be seen, mortality in the Turkmen Republic increased considerably in all main hospital departments. The highest increase was for psychiatric patients and for children suffering from diseases of the ear, nose, and throat, and from tuberculosis. This contingent of patients are most affected by the unfavorable conditions caused by an earthquake. In addition, the general social and economic state of a country and the existence or not of a plan for dealing with natural disasters all affect the overall result. During the early postwar period the situation in the USSR was especially difficult. No planned, effective system for dealing with the effects of earthquakes existed.

In summary then, the public health consequences of earthquakes are characterized by:

1. Massive traumatic injuries incurred during the short beginning period of the quake, and the effects of stress; among the injured, women and children prevail
2. Peculiar ratio of killed to injured, varying from 1:0.3 to 1:15; traumatic injuries prevailing over other disease in the initial period (95%)
3. Prevalence of fractures of the extremities (17%), skull traumas (15%–37%), and soft tissue wounds with hemorrhages (32%) among the severely wounded; minor wounds to the extremities (60%) and to the head among the slightly wounded
4. Increase in cardiovascular disease and aggravation of the course of disease; hypertensive cardiocerebral disease complicated by infarction, disturbances in cerebral circulation, and increased mortality; more neuroses and other psychiatric illnesses observed during the second period of the earthquake
5. Spread of infectious diseases, especially intestinal (typhoid, dysentery), children's (diphtheria, measles, whooping cough, scarlet fever), malaria, transmissible tropical diseases, observed at later stages

Public Health Consequences of Tsunami

The word "tsunami" is of Japanese origin, meaning "big wave in the harbor." Tsunami are caused by the upward or downward shifting of sections of the ocean bed, usually following strong underwater or coastal earthquakes. Sometimes they are caused by volcanic eruptions and other tectonic processes. These suddenly appearing, devastating waves reflect dramatic changes in sea bed topography, i.e., descent and ascent of rock masses along the soil breaks and sinking of noncondensed material. Tsunami are the greatest natural disaster of all.

The problem of fighting tsunami is a current one. Solutions have been far from satisfactory, especially with regard to protection and administration of aid, in particular medical aid, which is mostly provided after considerable delay.

Following the earthquake which took place on September 23, 1923, the bed of the Sagami Sea (Japan) underwent incredible transformations. Most of it rose 450 m, but certain sections sank 720 m, resulting in a tremendous amplitude of more than 1 km. The direct effect of such transformation on the ocean surface is drastic, disturbing its natural balance over a vast area [118, 201, 233, 236]. Tsunami can reach 100 km in length and have a period ranging from 2 to 200 min [235]. They are not noticed on board ship, but on approaching the coast they become a series of steep waves with tremendous damaging force.

In planning for protection and aid to the population, the following must be taken into consideration:

1. The intensity of the tsunami's impact on the coast depends on the intensity of the preceding earthquake and the depth of its epicenter, on the distance between the epicenter and the coastline, and on the depth of the ocean at the epicenter of the tsunami
2. The speed with which the tsunami spreads from its origin to the coast is proportional to GH, where H is the ocean depth and G the gravitational force acceleration; this value reaches 700–1000 km/h depending on the ocean depth
3. The height of the wave increases in bays, with peaks narrowing in the direction of the depth and in the river valleys; in wide bays with narrow entrances the waves lose height
4. The height of the wave increases when the wave passes over underwater mountain range and decreases over underwater valleys [224]

According to the Japanese scientist Miesi Hisasi, preventive measures are needed in regions characterized by the following features:

a) U- and V-shaped bays,
b) islands situated near to each other, and
c) the low areas of capes [169].

Tsunami are a natural phenomenon predetermined by the earth's tectonic evolution and cannot be prevented; the reason for their appearance cannot be eliminated. However, the complex of the above-stated features and knowledge of tsunamogenic zones do, to a certain extent, enable prediction of the condition under which they will occur and their consequences. Recurrent tsunami can be expected in places of frontal island arc prominence or jut where previous earthquakes with tsunami have taken place [153]. With regard to the damage they cause, sea waves are similar to the waves that result from dam bursts.

There are also tsunami which are caused by meteorological factors; these are long waves resulting from cyclone movement in medium latitudes. The low pressure at the center of a cyclone has a suction on the water surface. The water begins to rise and then, under gravitational force, becomes a huge wave. Other waves may be caused by the fast drifting of water into the coast, a bay, or a delta owing to a strong, one-directional wind [172]. Meteorological tsunami are especially devastating in connection with typhoons. Poniavin [199] identifies the meteorologically determinded tsunami as the cause of the Leningrad floods, brought on by strong winds affecting the Baltic Sea surface and by fast, abnormal changes in atmospheric pressure.

Tsunami are encountered mostly in the Pacific Ocean zone, with 80% of them appearing on its periphery [236], striking Alaska, Kamchatka, the Japanese and Hawaiian Islands, and the west coast of Canada. In the USSR, tsunami are registered mostly on Kamchatka, the Kuril, and the Komandor Islands. The average height of tsunami striking the Pacific coastline of the USSR ranges from 10 to 18 m, depending on relief features; the outside range is between 1 and 37 m [236]. Weak tsunami have taken place and could recur in the seismoactive regions of the Black and Caspian Seas, the Arctic Ocean, and Lake Baikal. USSR territories subject to tsunami of seismic and meteorological origin are shown in Fig. 8 [32].

On the eastern coast of Kamchatka and the Kuril Islands, regions determined vulnerable to tsunami are Kronotsky, Shipunsky, Piratkov, Povorotnij, Kamchatsky, Kamenistij, Storozh, Morzhevaja and Listvenichnaja bays, and the Malo-Kurilsky and Vtoroj-Kurilsky Straits [107, 120, 219, 236]. The Kamchatka and Kuril Island coasts are susceptible mainly in the zone of the Kuril-Kamchatsky cavity, relatively close to the coast. Because of the depth of the cavity a tsunami reaches the coast 20–30 min after the beginning of an earthquake [134]. The central part of the Kuril arc is in the most dangerous situation; it takes only 10–15 min for tsunami to reach it. In a better position are the islands of Shikotan (15–25 min), Iturup (20–25 min), Paramushir (30–35 min), and Kunashir (more than 60 min) [233]. These islands are included in the Sakhalin administrative region.

Tsunami attacks are frequent in the United States as well. For the period 1946–1964, seven tsunami, with waves reaching 7 m, were registered in Crescent City, California. The most devastating occurred on March 28, 1964 [154].

Fig. 8. Areas in the USSR that are subject to tsunami of seismic and meteorologic origin

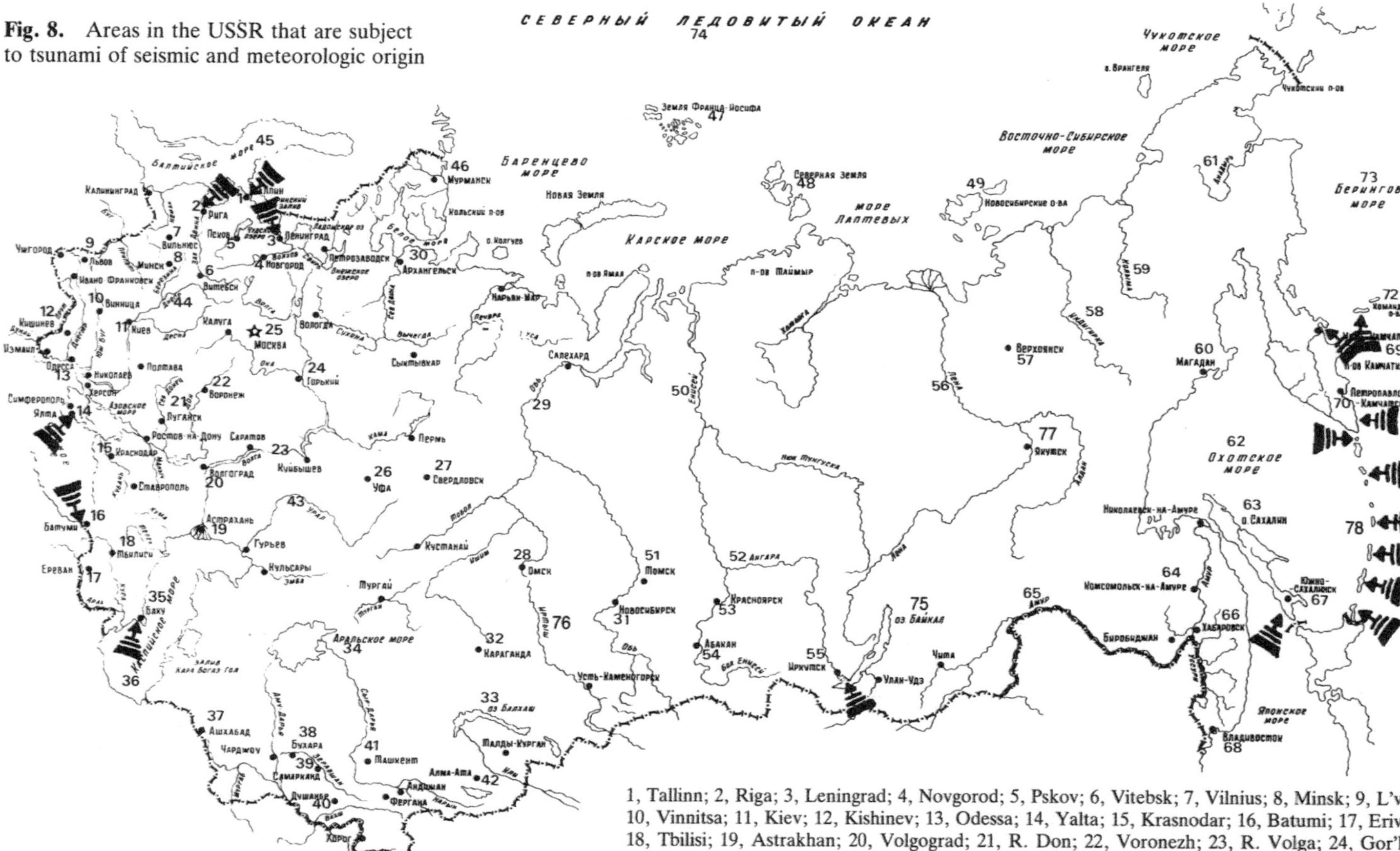

1, Tallinn; 2, Riga; 3, Leningrad; 4, Novgorod; 5, Pskov; 6, Vitebsk; 7, Vilnius; 8, Minsk; 9, L'vov; 10, Vinnitsa; 11, Kiev; 12, Kishinev; 13, Odessa; 14, Yalta; 15, Krasnodar; 16, Batumi; 17, Erivan; 18, Tbilisi; 19, Astrakhan; 20, Volgograd; 21, R. Don; 22, Voronezh; 23, R. Volga; 24, Gor'kiy; 25, Moscow; 26, Ufa; 27, Sverdlovsk; 28, Omsk; 29, R. Ob'; 30, Archangelsk; 31, Novosibirsk; 32, Karaganda; 33, Lake Balkhash; 34, Aral Sea; 35 Baku; 36, Caspian Sea; 37, Ashkhabad; 38, Bukhara; 39 Samarkand; 40, Dushanbe; 41, Tashkent; 42, Alma-Ata; 43, R. Ural; 44, R. Dnieper; 45, Baltic Sea; 46, Murmansk; 47, Franz Josef Land; 48, Severnaya Zemliya; 49, New Siberian Is.; 50, R. Yenisey; 51, Tomsk; 52, R. Angara; 53, Krasnoyarsk; 54, Abakan; 55, Irkutsk; 56, R. Lena; 57, Verkhoyansk; 58, R. Indigirka; 59, R. Kolyma; 60, Magadan; 61, R. Anadyr; 62, Sea of Okhotsk; 63, Sakhalin Island; 64, Komsomolsk na Amure; 65, R. Amur; 66, Khabarovsk; 67, Yuzhno-Sakhalinsk; 68, Vladivostok; 69, Kamchatka Peninsula; 70, Petropavlovok-Kamchatskiy; 71, Ust'-Kamchatsk; 72, Komandorskiye Is.; 73, Bering Sea; 74, Arctic Ocean; 75, Lake Baykal; 76, R. Irtysh; 77, Yakutsk; 78, Kuril Isl.

Objective data on the above mentioned areas and events can help in the following:

1. Planning for prevention, protection, and provision of aid in susceptible regions
2. Estimation of available resources and their allocation for efficient handling of the effects of a tsunami attack
3. Settling up of observation facilities and information services to warn the population and respective authorities of approaching tsunami

Tsunami information services in the USSR, the United States, and Japan are in constant cooperation with one another. This is an example of international solidarity, which must be the basis for a universal warning system on natural disasters. Tsunami of seismic and meteorological origin have struck such countries as Bangladesh, Greece, Indonesia, India, Italy, Canada, Morocco, New Zealand, Portugal, the United States, Turkey, and the Philippines. To this list can be added Australia, the Netherlands, France, the Federal Republic of Germany, and countries in Latin America, which have suffered the grave consequences of dam breaks and blocked mountain lakes, resembling the effects of tsunami.

Tsunami are also predetermined by anthropogenic factors, connected with the international ecological crisis. We cannot overlook the occurrence of underwater atomic explosions. Kahn and Wiener [126] discuss the possibility that tsunami have been caused during the past two decades by atomic testing with military aims.

As shown in Fig. 9, an underwater atomic explosion can cause huge waves, similar to those caused by the eruption of island volcanoes. The American Baker Test is an

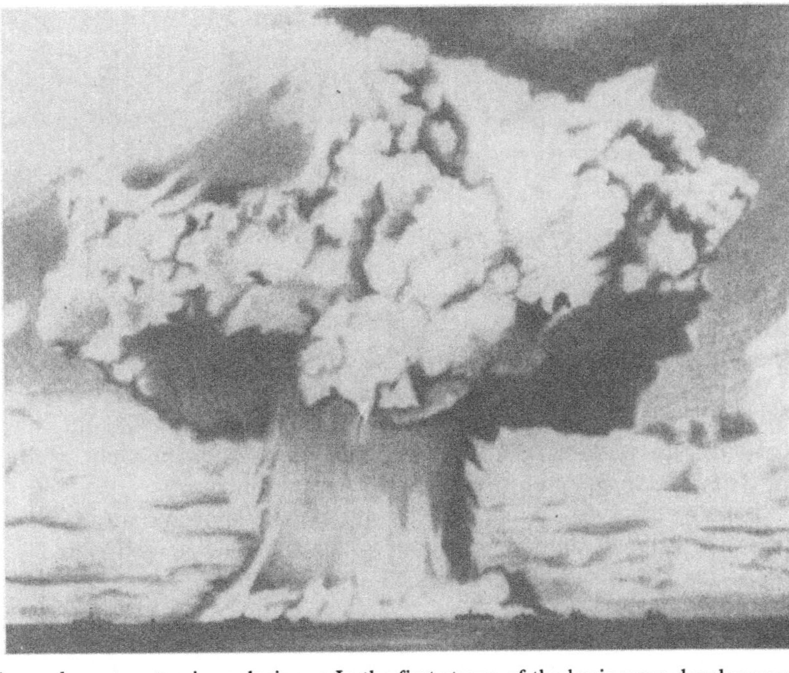

Fig. 9a, b. An underwater atomic explosion. **a** In the first stages of the basic wave development. **b** see p. 32

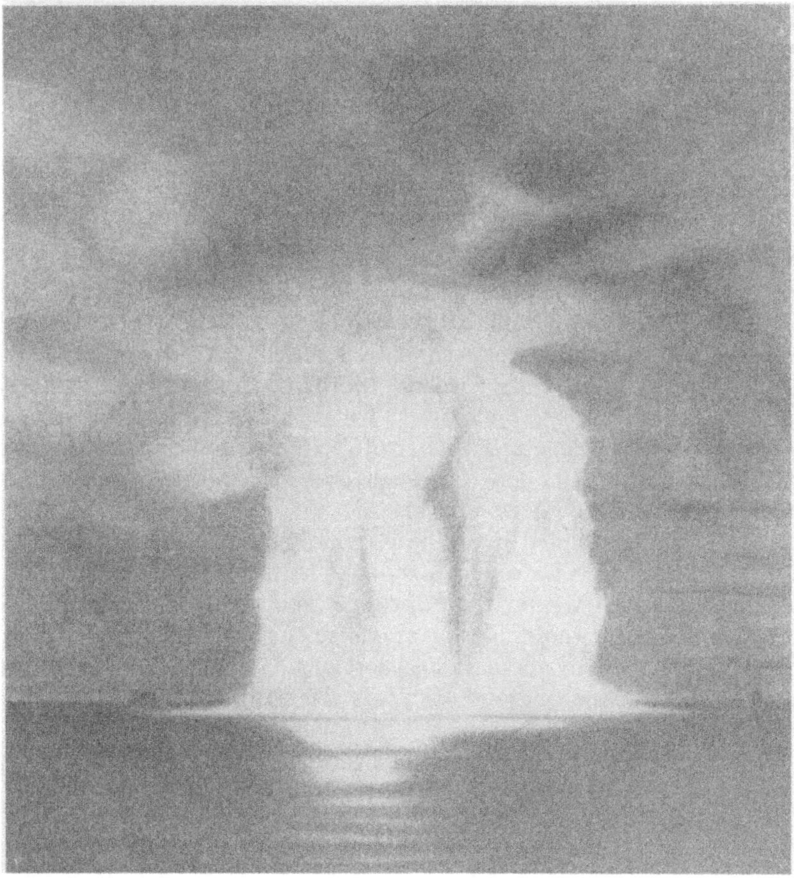

Fig. 9. **b** The underwater atomic explosion

example of an underwater explosion in shallow waters (about 15 m) equivalent to 100 000 tons of TNT. The first sea wave it caused extended for 540 m from the epicenter, in 15 s. Its height was 54 m, the pressure reached 80 kg/cm^2, and its duration was 0.01 s. Pressure can reach a maximun of 150 kg/cm^2. An aerial shockwave also occurs [188].

Missiles and bombs dropped during a military crises can create flood zones. Military actions can also destroy dikes, dams, sluices, and other hydrotechnical contructions. Although such actions deliberate tactics of military strategy, events may develop to the point where things get out of control.

Tsunami cannot be prevented, but the population can be protected by

a) construction of autonomous underground shelters (dugouts) and

b) evacuation to safe, higher areas.

Early warning of the approaching disaster is of the greatest importance. The most outstanding sign is a considerable retreat of the ocean coincident with low tide. This is the first sign of an approaching wave, which follows in 10–15 min. The ocean's

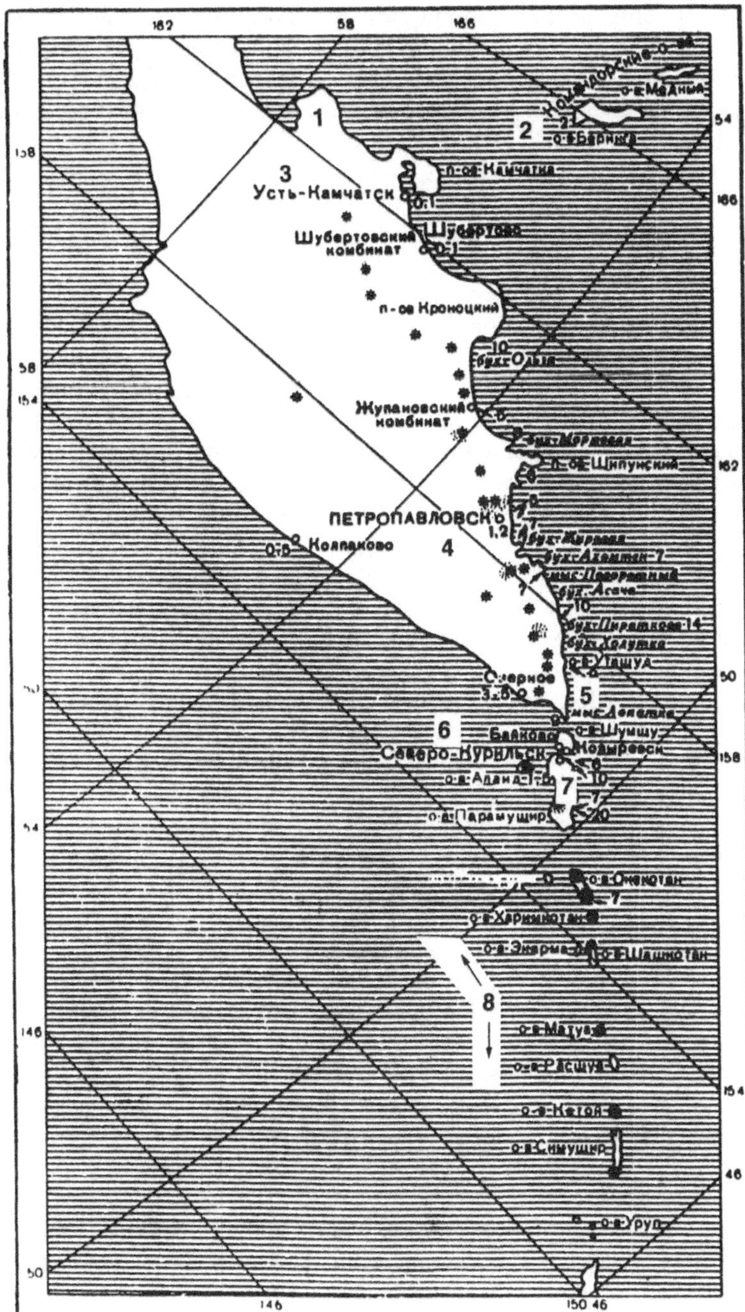

Fig. 10. Kuril-Kamchatka tsunami 1952. The numbers in smaller print indicate the height of tsunami waves (m), the cluster of dots show the area endangered by the volcanic eruptions, the stars represent active volcanoes: 1, Cape Dzernoi; 2, Komandorskiye Is.; 3, Ust'Kamchatsk; 4, Petropavlovsk-Kamchatskiy; 5, Cape Lopatka; 6, Severo-Kuril'sk; 7, Paramushir Is.; 8, Kuril Is

retreat continues for 8–35 min, and the shore becomes bare for hundreds of meters. The greater the retreat, the stronger is the coming tsunami. Special devices, called mareographs, register changes in the ocean level near the coast and are used to detect these waves. Hydroacoustical devices detect waves caused by underwater volcanic eruptions [134].

The tsunami which lashed Kamchatka and the Kuril Islands during the night of November 4–5, 1952 was preceded by a magnitude-7 earthquake (magnitude 10 at its epicenter). The waves reached a height of 20 m, averaging heights of 7–8 m along 1000 km of coastline [219] (see Fig. 10).

According to information from eyewitnesses, 45 min after the beginning of the earthquake a loud roaring sound resembling cannonade was heard from the ocean. The coast was hit by a gigantic wave bearing sand, silt, and debris. In a few minutes the water retreated, taking with it the remains of destroyed buildings. Silence came, and hundreds of meters out from the shore, one could see the sea bed. Fifteen minutes later another wave came, exceeding the first one in strength and height. A few minutes later came the third, this one weaker than its predecessors. Here and there whirlpools appeared, remnants of buildings and small boats spinning in them with incredible speed. People caught in the whirlpools drowned immediately [218].

A Tsunami wave is capable of traveling thousands of miles while preserving sufficient energy to be 5 m high as it hits the coast. Tsunami have been known to have reached a height of more than 40 m, flooding and damaging the coastal plans 2 and more miles inland. On April 1, 1946 an 11-m-high tsunami was caused by an earthquake which took place in the region of Unimak Island, in the Aleutians. It reached Hawaii (a distance of 3700 km away) in 5 h, with an average speed of 740 km/h. Three huge waves, striking mainly Oahu Island, followed each other at 20-min intervals [224, 225].

Figure 11 gives a general visual idea of the consequences of these devastating waves. Press reports on the tsunami which struck Chile on May 22, 1960 estimated the length of damaged coastline at >1000 km. The waves retreated back into the Pacific, destroying the towns of Puerto Saavedro, Puerto Monti, and Ankua, and revealing kilometers of ocean bottom.

On several occasions in Japan and the Hawaiian Islands waves have reached a height of 10 m, on the Kuril Islands 5–7 m, and on Kamchatka 3–5 m. Having studied wave height in relat on to damage done by tsunami, the Japanese scientist Imamura (cited in Poniavin [199]) elaborated a classification of these two parameters (Table 10). Tsunami in groups III, IV, and V seriously affect public health and safety. In cases of seismically caused tsunami, one must consider the injurious of the

Table 10. Classification of tsunami (Imamura)

Group	Degree	Wave height (m)	Damage
I	0	1	Constructions on coast unscathed
II	1	2	Houses destroyed, small ships thrown against coast
III	2	4–6	Houses destroyed, heavy damage to husbandry
IV	3	10–20	Heavy damage along 400 km of coastline
V	4	30	Catastrophic damage along 500 km of coastline

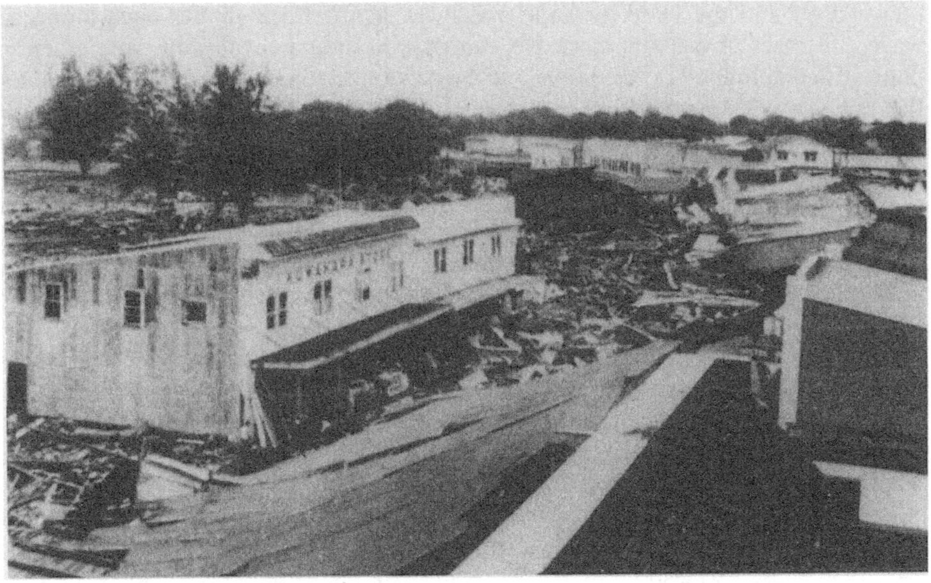

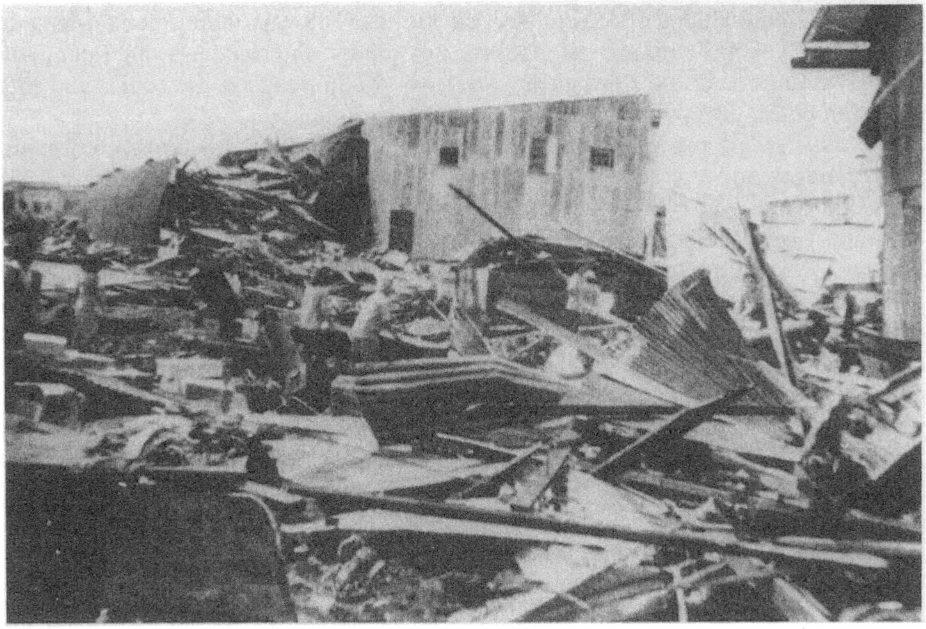

Fig. 11. Consequences of tsunami in one of the Hawaiian Islands [225]

quake itself and the hydrodynamic and hydrostatic effects of the devastating sea waves. In cases of tsunami caused by underwater atomic explosions, the extent of damage is determined by the impact of the wave, the subsequent surface waves, and the radioactive compounds of the atomic bomb. Atomic explosions are especially dangerous for the populations of coastal cities. They may damage dams on big rivers and the resulting floods may damage cities and towns downriver.

When a tsunami strikes an area it causes devastation and many deaths in a short period of time. This is a relatively rare phenomenon, and its effect is local. The devastating wave which appeared after the 1908 earthquake at Messina washed houses away from the coastline in Reggio; they were simply severed from the land. Many people drowned in the wave [103]. In 1923, three successive waves damaged the eastern coastline of Kamchatka. They reached heights of 6 m, and struck a roughtly 480 km length of coastline between Khalaktyrka and Ust-Kamchatsk. The waves tore off a layer of coastal ice 2 m thick. In the low-lying area near Semiachik, the ice layer was thrown more than a kilometer into the ocean, and the whole lowland was flooded [187].

Tsunami are frightening, and lack of knowledge about them aggravates the difficult situation that results. The earthquake followed by a tsunami on November 4–5, 1952 caused widespread panic on Kamchatka and the Kuril Islands. Terrified people ran from their houses half naked, and when the quake was over they returned, unaware of the coming tsunami. The retreating ocean was sign enough of the calamity to come; unfortunately, most people were ignorant of its significance. Most of the populations of Severo Kurilsk, Bukhta Kitovaja, and other settlements were killed. People trapped in houses sunk under the water, swam along the ceilings, trying to escape through the windows. Many reached the roofs, and then telegraph poles. A few managed to reach higher ground.

The wave swept away all the buildings, leaving behind only the concrete foundations. Bridges and the stone decking of highways were torn away. A large, self-propelled barge which was on the river at the time was thrown 2 km. In Bukhta Kitovaja, where the wave reached a height of 20 m, all constructions were washed into the ocean. Only one wall of the power station and a generator mounted on a concrete floor remained. Half a kilometer from a house situated 12–13 m above sea level, a steamer was found, thrown up out of the ocean. Fig. 12 offers an idea of the power of this tsunami [218]. Settlements not situated high enough along the eastern coastline of Kamchatka and the Kuril Islands were destroyed. Hardest hit were those along the lowest banks of the First Kuril Strait, the eastern bank of Paramushir Island, and the narrow, wedge-shaped bays of southeast Kamchatka [233].

A similar picture of damage was reported in Chile (1960). Table 11 illustrates the magnitude of damage caused by catastrophic tsunami. They appear suddenly, and frequently are relatively localized. As can be seen from the table, any protective measures undertaken have had little effect, and the extent of damages today appears to be as great as it was in the past.

The damaging factors of tsunami determine the structure of injuries, as shown in Table 12, compiled from various sources [118, 147, 199, and others]. The table shows a high percentage of people killed or lost, i.e., washed into the sea and drowned. This contingent of victims comprises from 10% to 60% of the total

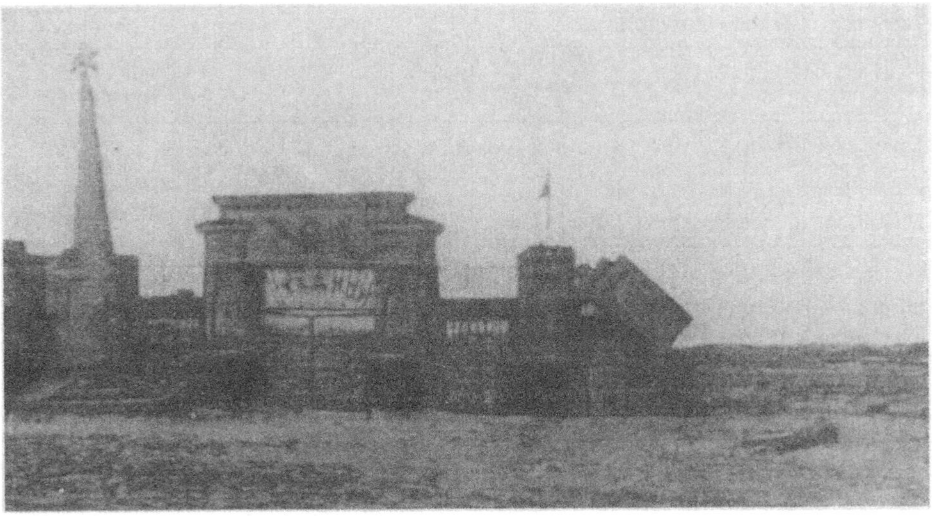

Fig. 12. Cement gates of a stadium partially destroyed by a tsunami; the gates are perpendicular to the direction in which the wave moved

Table 11. Description and effects of selected tsunami

Location	Origin	Wave height (m)	Fatalities	Comment
Bay of Bengal, 1732 [39]	Meteorologic	13	300 000	
Kyushu Island (Shimabara Bay, Japan), May 21, 1792 [224]	Landslide after earthquake	–	15 000	3 large waves
St. Petersburg, 1824 [32]	Meteorologic	–	569	4 000 people fell ill
Japan, 1869 [118]	Seismic	30	27 122	10 000 houses washed away
Song Da Islands, 1883 [218]	Underwater volcanic eruption	36	36 000	
Galveston, Texas, USA, 900 [224]	Storms	–	6 000	Sea rose as a wall
Ito settlement, Japan, 1923 [215]	Seismic	–	14 000	
Kamchatka, Kuril Islands (Shumsu, Paramushir, Onekotan, and others), 1952 [218, 219]	Seismic	10–20	–	Severokurilsk and other settlements destroyed
Ionian Islands, Greece, 1953 [137]	Seismic	–	Hundreds	Port of Veti destroyed
Hamburg, FRG, 1962 [111]	Meteorologic	–	500	
Islands of the Ganges Delta, the Bay of Bengal, Bangladesh, and India, 1970[a]	Hurricane	10	300 000 to 2 000 000	

[a] French radio and press

Table 12. Casualties of tsunami

Place and date	Injured	Killed/lost	Ratio of injured to killed/lost
Japan, 1896	9 247	27 122	1:2.9
Italy, 1908	1 650	1 600	1:1
City of Hilo, 1960	282	61	1:0.2
Hawaii, Maui, Molokai, Oahu, Kauai, 1960	163	159	1:1

number killed by a tsunami. The ratio between wounded and killed or missing may vary from 1:0.2 to 1:3, depending to a certain extent on the effectiveness of rescue operations.

Among the wounded, injuries to the trunk and the extremities prevail, caused by impact with parts of buildings destroyed by the earthquake and borne by the tsunami or floating on the flood waters. Most of the drowned are women and children. As in the case of earthquakes, this can be explained by the fact that women and children are more helpless in undertaking protective and rescue measures on their own, and are more vulnerable to the effects of stress. This was documented in Leningrad after the meteorologically caused tsunami of September 23, 1924 [292].

In the next stage, people face the disturbances of local ecological conditions, in particular in the course of general and infectious diseases. There is an apparent interdependence between sea storms, the general situation of stress, the increase in humidity and cold (i.e., environmental conditions concurrent with tsunami), and a proliferation of asthma attacks [263].

Among people rescued from drowning the percentage with serious pneumonia is especially high. Frequently, death is caused by overcooling as a result of being in the water for a long time. According to a report by the Pacific Sakhalin medical institutions attended to water transport, the causes of death among passengers on ships hit by a tsunami off the Kuril Islands in 1952 were distributed as follows: pneumonia, 18%, overcooling, 6%. This tsunami mostly struck the Sakhalin region, on November 4–5. The morbidity and mortality reported from this administrative area for 1952–1953 provide an assessment of the public health consequences of tsunami. Taking the number of patients delivered to medical institutions in the Sakhalin region in 1952 as 100%, this figure is estimated at 124% for 1953. The changes in the character of diseases, and the reasons for increases in morbidity and mortality are shown in Fig. 13 and 14, based on reports from the health institutions of the region [32]. After the tsunami attack (i.e., by the end of 1952) there was an increased number of patients suffering eye diseases, gynecological disorders, psychoses and neuroses, internal and infectious diseases, and diseases of the ear, nose, and throat (see Fig. 13).

Those with traumatic injuries were evacuated immediately after the calamity (i.e., after November 5) to the town of Yuzhno Sakhalinsk and to the mainland. Though the number of patients requiring surgery did not increase drastically in 1953 (104.3%), mortality in this group reached 113.7% owing to the specific character of the injuries and the course of the diseases. Increases in mortality were also registered among gynecologic patients (112.1%) and especially among children with infectious diseases (159%).

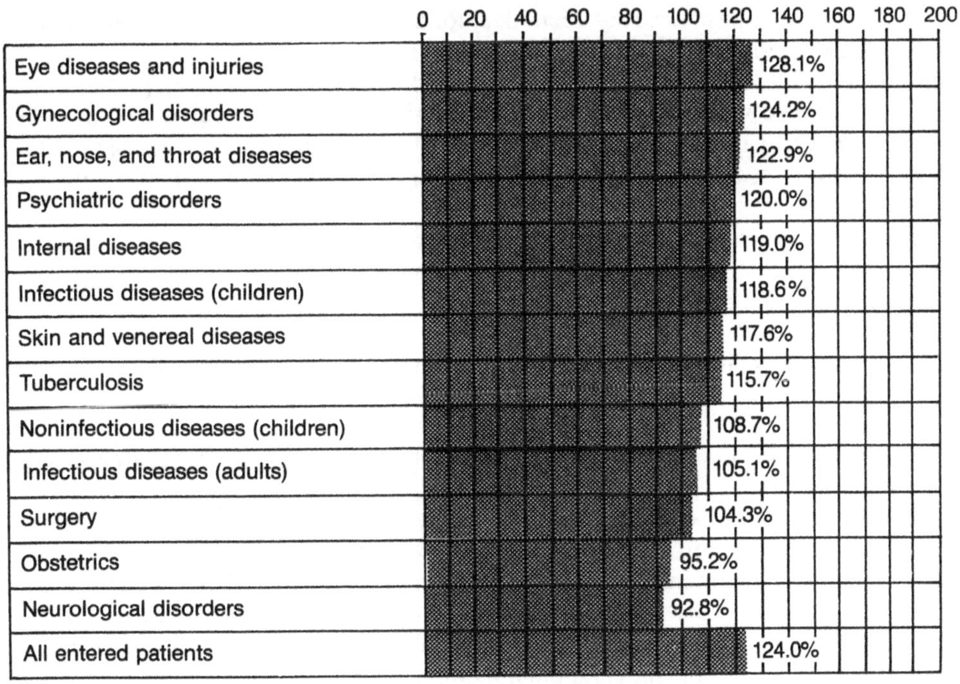

Fig. 13. Morbidity of patients' entering the hospitals of the Sakhalin region in 1953 in comparison with 1952 (1952 taken as 100%)

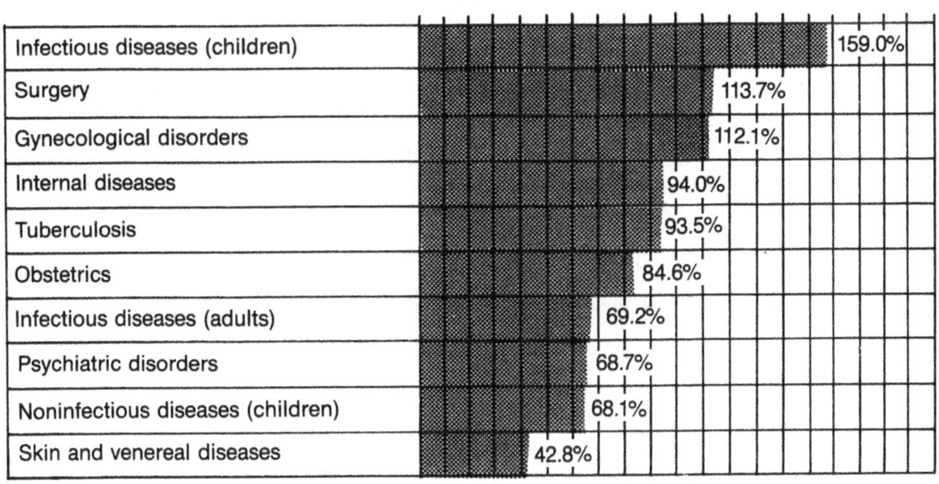

Fig. 14. Mortality in the hospitals of the Sakhalin region in 1953 in comparison with 1952 (1952 taken as 100%)

Although I do not possess sufficient data for a deep and comprehensive analysis of the reasons for the stated increase in mortality, it appears justified to connect it with the unfavorable environmental conditions, which badly affect the provision of medical aid, and with the character of the injuries themselves, caused as they were by the impact of the tsunami. It seems instructive to consider the dynamics of the way in which some of these diseases developed – evidently promoted by the particular conditions.

The following problems are directly attributable to the effects of a tsunami attack:

a) various types of traumatic injuries,
b) overcooling and increased humidity,
c) emotional stress,
d) unfavorable environmental conditions causing both decreased resistance and the epidemic spread of disease.

The migration of a large portion of the population of a stricken area also plays a role in the spread of disease.

The 1952 tsunami caused the deaths of many people in the Sakhalin region. The absence of planning for such an emergency, the remoteness of the territory struck, and the difficult communication conditions of the area hampered an effective rescue operation. The problem of providing medical aid remained unsolved; the Yuzhno Sakhalinsk medical team, sent to provide qualifed assistance to the rescue teams, in fact remained on the sidelines and did not directly participate in the rescue activities. The situation made systematic medical documentation impossible. Researchers are obliged to limit themselves to data related to the criteria of general medicine, foregoing the indispensable data on the specific situation.

Table 13 gives the incidence of some disorders; it was compiled from data provided by the Sakhalin regional authorities and processed by the Scientific Methodological Bureau of Public Health Statistics of the Russian Soviet Federated Socialist Republic [293]. The morbidity for 1952 in the Sakhalin region is compared with the rates for the Republic as a whole, and, as can be seen, the indicence of traumas and pneumonia in 1952 was 1.5–1.6 times higher in the Sakhalin region than in the Republic overall. This index corresponds to the expected structure of injuries from tsunami, as well as to the anticipated prevalence of pneumonia complications. This latter fact is also predetermined by climatic conditions. During the Second World War, 18.7% of wounded Soviet soldiers had pneumonia. The highest incidence of pneumonia was on the northern fronts (17,5%), the lowest on the southern fronts (6%) [223].

Table 13. Nosology of first admission to hospital, RSFSR and Sakhalin region, 1952 (all values in %)[a]

Reason for admission	RSFSR	Sakhalin region	Increase
Trauma	6.3	9.4	50
Pneumonia	0.9	1.4	60
Skin disease	6.7	7.7	15

[a] Data processed by Bureau of Public Health Statistics, RSFSR [352]

Table 14. Mortality of pneumonia patients treated at home (%)

	Croupous pneumonia		Other forms of pneumonia	
	1951	1952	1951	1952
Sakhalin region	24.4	36.4	19.5	42.8
RSFSR as a whole	30.1	22.9	35.3	38.3

Overcooling of the body, combined with increased humidity and late arrival of medical aid, caused the high mortality of patients with pneumonia (all forms) who were under home regime (Table 14). In the Sakhalin administrative region in 1952 the mortality of patients treated at home increased drastically. For cases of croupous pneumonia it was 1.5 times higher than in the precious year, and for other types it was twice as high. The extreme environmental situation caused by the tsunami badly influences emergency medical aid, public health activities, and evacuation. Treatment and evacuation of people with traumatic injuries that render them nontransportable is especially difficult.

The mortality for the injured who get no qualified treatment and remain at home is very high. According to the Scientific Methodological Public Health Bureau of the RSFSR Ministry of Health, for those treated at home in the Sakhalin region it was 11.9% in 1951 and 40.8% in 1952. In the Russian Republic in general the figures were 6.2%, 1951 and 7.8%, 1952. That is to say, the mortality from traumas among the injured who stayed at home was 3.4 times higher in 1952 than in 1951.

The effects of tsunami are bad as well for the contingent of the population suffering from chronic diseases. Their course becomes complicated and the need for hospitalization increases (Table 15). The percentage of patients with chronic illnesses and the complications to their illnesses increases drastically in 1952. Particularly among cardiovascular patients, both at home and hospitalized, there was increased mortality. The neuropsychological factor is significant here, for these people suffered both the stress of their illness and the stress of the natural disaster simultaneously.

Table 15. Patients with chronic diseases, Sakhalin region, 1951–1953 (%) [352]

	1951	1952	1953	Increase (%)
A. Hospital admissions [293]				
Gastric and duodenum ulcer	4.1	6.1		50
Liver and biliary tract disease	3.9	5.0		30
Diseases of urinary system	4.9	7.4		50
B. Died at home[a]				
Cerebro vascular sclerosis	4.8	75.0	33.3	
Cardiac valve diseases	20.7	36.1	not reported	
Myocardial diseases	48.3	54.4	50.0	
C. Died in hospital[a]				
Myocardial diseases	3.7	5.7	7.2	
Hypertension	1.7	3.8	2.3	

[a] As proportion of total deaths from these diseases (%)

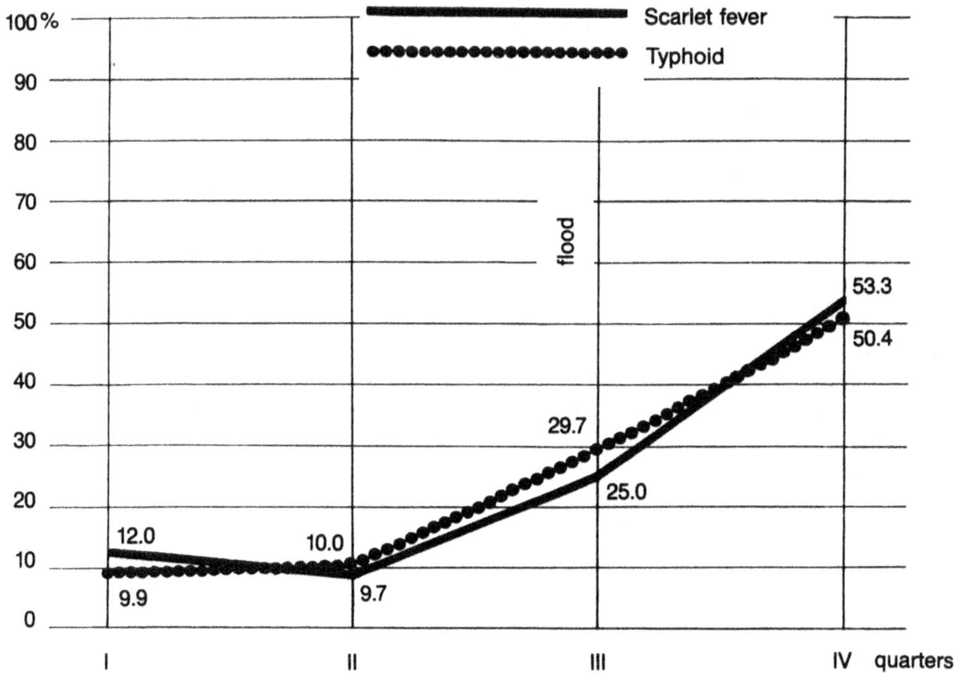

Fig. 15. Incidence of scarlet fever and typhoid in connection with the Leningrad flood (1924)

Nonfunctioning water and sewage systems and the need for mass evacuation of the population promote the spread of infectious diseases. To a large extent, this is predetermined by the epidemiological and public situation that existed before the disaster, for which the local authorities are responsible. In Leningrad, even before the flood of September 23, 1924 (caused by a meteorological tsunami), there was a high incidence of scarlet fever and typhoid. However, a further increase was observed after the flood. Fig. 15, based on reports by the Leningrad health authorities, demonstrates this [32, 294]. In the third quarter and the following fourth quarter the number of scarlet fever cases increases 3.6-fold; the corresponding figures for typhoid show a fourfold increase. Analysis shows that these increases were due to mass migration of the population, made homeless by the flood, and deteriorating sanitary conditions caused by disturbances to the water supply and sewage systems.

Table 16. Number of cases of infectious disease, Vasilievsky Island, 1924

	First quarter	Second quarter	Third quarter	Fourth quarter	Total
Typhoid	8	4	28	40	80
Scarlet fever	65	46	85	178	374
Dysentery	4	8	86	18	116

The Moskovsko Narvsky district of the city had a population of 240 000. This area was the most damaged by the flood. An epidemic of sarlet fever broke out there and a number of schools were closed [295]. Vasilievsky Island, which was in the flood zone, was badly affected by the worsening epidemiological and sanitary conditions.

As can be seen in Table 16 [296], there was a considerable increase in typhoid and scarlet fever cases in the third and fourth quarters of the year (the tsunami occurred on September 23). Especially high was the incidence of dysentery in the third quarter. The situation I observed on Kamchatka after the meteorological tsunami of November 1957 was similar. According to a report by the hospital of the Oktiabr administrative district of the Kamchatka region, the increase in the number of cases of dysentery was 44%, the main reason being the pollution of soil and water after the attack.

Table 17. Origin and consequences of tsunami, and organized protective response

Origin
Seismic
Volcanic
Meteorologic
Anthropogenic
Hydroelectric plant, ecological or other disturbances (not depending on war)
Underwater atomic explosions or other explosions (during wartime)
General injurious factors
Hydrodynamic and hydrostatic effects of waves
Destruction borne by waves
Local ecological changes
Specific injurious factors
Preceding earthquake
Cyclone, storm
Air shock wave
Radioactive particles
Type of casualties
Immediate
Drownings
Traumatic injuries
Subsequent
Increased general morbidity, caused mainly by rapid cooling and heightened humidity
Increased infectious morbidity, mainly intestinal and children's diseases
Radioactive injuries and injuries caused by air shock wave (underwater atomic explosions)
Method of protection
Observation and efficient information processing of tsunami and mudflows
Control and observation of hydroelectric constructions, reservoirs, and blocked mountain lakes
Placement of settlements on elevated areas, construction of protective dams, breakwater piers, programmed tree planting
Timely evacuation of population
Efficient equipping of autonomous shelters

Table 17 gives the general characteristics of tsunami. We can see that their very nature require us to provide for the following:

1. More precise definition of tsunamogenic zones, according to causes, conditions, potential force, and damages
2. Planning for provision of aid, especially medical, taking into consideration the peculiarities of the situation and the structure of injuries at the initial stage and later on
3. Cooperation between tsunami observation and information services
4. Safety measures for hydrotechnical constructions, mountain reservoirs, etc. that are part of the local environmental sanitation activities
5. A plan to evacuate the population when a tsunami threatens

Practical implementation of these propositions is difficult and entails considerable expense. It is dependent on the socioeconomic situation of the country in question, and in most countries vulnerable to tsunami this is not optimal. However, to minimize the devastating effects of tsunami there ist no other alternative.

Public Health Consequences of Floods

With regard to the consequences, including those for public health, floods are the most frequent and severe natural disaster. The causes of floods are
a) natural and therefore unavoidable, or
b) anthropogenic, and thus avoidable by sanitation of the environment, and supervision and control of construction activities, hydroelectric buildings, and other industrial complexes which could cause damage to the environment.

Floods are directly connected with
a) prolonged, abundant rain or cloudbursts or fast melting of snow and ice because of a drastic temperature increase;
b) mudflows and tsunami, of both seismic and meteorological origin;
c) ecological disturbances, as well as failures in construction and operation of hydroelectric or other such projects.

Floods frequently occur after earthquakes have caused breaks in mountain lakes, reservoirs, or dams.

With regard to the USSR, about one million km^2 (about 5% of the total territory) is susceptible to annual flooding [152]. Most dangerous are the rivers Amu-Daria, Amur, Dnieper, Dniester, Desna, Danube, and Ural, and the Azov Sea. In the 22 million km^2 covered by the USSR, about 10 000 large and medium-sized rivers flow [152]. Their constantly increasing pollution and environmental pollution in general make water more and more a medium for the spread of intestinal diseases. This is all the more true when there is a flood. According to Vakhula [256], in the USSR in 1976–1977, 58 salmonella cultures of ten serotypes and *Shigella flexneri* were extracted from water tested from open reservoirs and sewage. It was also determined that in two cases of acute intestinal disease the agent transferring the infection was the polluted river water and possibly the drinking water from the water supply system. The situation is similar in other countries: In China, samples taken from 82 rivers and adjacent areas showed pollution in 45 cases [297].

Unsatisfactory water supply systems and the vulnerability of the population to infection caused by polluted water is a situation common to many countries. According to an Asian representative at the XXII World Health Assembly, 60% of morbidity and 40% of mortality in his country were the result of infections transfered by water, and 90% of the rural population (comprising about 72% of that country's total) suffers from diseases caused by intestinal parasites. The water supply pipeline of this country serves less than 10% of the people [298].

Figure 16 shows the USSR territories which suffer recurring floods. The peculiarities of hydrography and the placing of settlements, hydroelectric stations and adjacent reservoirs make the European part of the USSR especially vulnerable to the damaging effects of floods. Losses incurred when 1 km^2 of land in this part of the Soviet Union is flooded can be valued at between 9 and 13 thousand rubles, while flooding of a similar area in the Asian part would result in losses valued only at 1.2–1.8 thousand rubles [41], i.e., eight times less.

The heaviest and most frequent floods happen in seismoactive and tsunamogenic areas, and in areas with the potential for mudflows. These areas are extremely vulnerable to a combination of natural disasters, which quite often complicate each other, increasing the damages. For example, when floods follow a drought the result is the biosocial disaster of famine.

Medunin [163] and Fiodorov [78] have written about the unsatisfactory treatment of ecological problems in the USSR. They note the need for scientific analysis of the transformation of natural conditions, in order to prevent the negative effects of both unintended and purposeful manipulations of the biosphere. They state that incorrect use of the soil and decimation of woodlands badly affect the landscape and promote floods of anthropogenic origin. Connected to this is the increasing soil erosion in the USSR, where, according to Armand [13], 52 million hectares have been washed of their soil and 4.5 million hectares are ravines. There is no movement to stop this process, which deprives the soil of its capacity to regulate itself.

Komarova [138] has observed disturbances in the water-protective function of mountain forests in the USSR and their diminishing role of water regulation. Floods now occur in Carpathia every 3–4 years, compared with, at 18 year intervals in the past; i.e., the frequency of floods there has increased almost fivefold. Deforestation aggravates and makes more frequent the catastrophic floods reported almost annually on the southwest slope of Sikhote-Alin, and the Ussuri and Suchan river watersheds [32].

In China, the enormous damage caused by the floods in the summer and fall of 1981 was closely connected to the cutting down of forests and destruction of the flora cover, creating an additional 27 000 km^2 of desert; about 1.5 million km^2 were affected by erosion. All this occured during the past 15 years [297].

Most floods in the USSR occur in the spring. They are most intensive in rivers that flow northward, where high water moving from the south meets melting ice. Towns situated on the northern river mouth, such as Arkhangelsk, Narian-Mar, and Salekhard, are particularly endangered.

In Central Asia, fast melting snow, and glaciers cause frequent summer floods. Floods in the Far East are caused by cloudburst rains and typhoons, which can appear at any season of the year.

The Leningrad floods are catastrophic. They are caused by winds forcing water from the Baltic Sea into the Neva River. In the course of the city's history, 226 such floods have been registered, most of them (85%) occurring in the autumn; 70% of theses floods began at night or in the morning, lasting on average for 26 h [268].

On the Dniester River (in Moldavia) the cycle of the floods occurring in the winter has reached 40 days. In summer 5–6 occur, but in some years the number was as high as 16, with a cycle ranging from 10 to 55 days [38]. Such floods often come suddenly, and generally last for 1–2 days, reaching their apogee in a few hours. In other cases

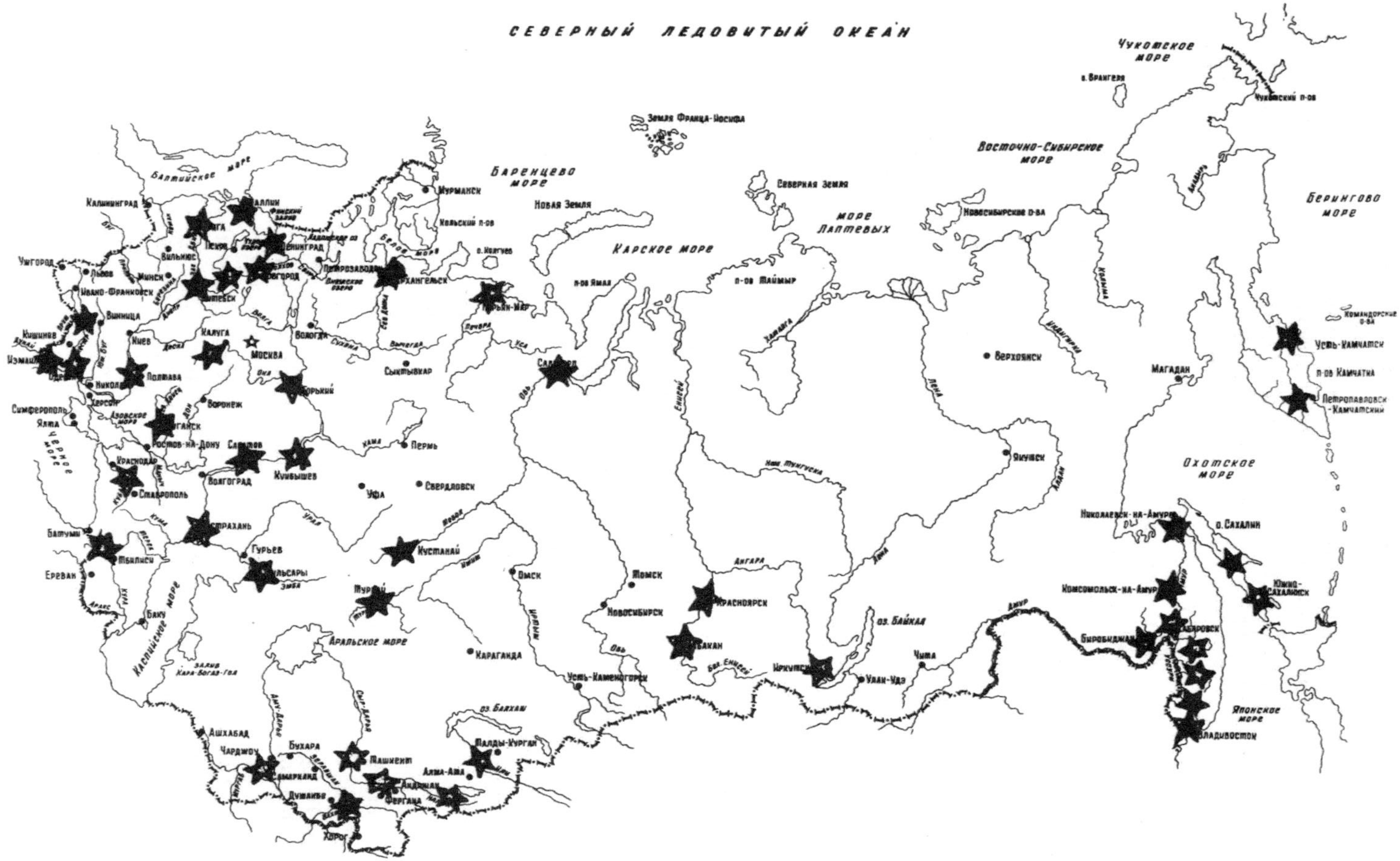

Fig. 16. USSR territories subject to floods

the water rises slowly, over the course of several days or even weeks. Such floods can last 2 months and more.

The overflow in the river mouth can cover an area 50–100 km in width and 500–1000 km along the riverbed. The water level rises 8–12 m and more. Rivers with unstable riverbeds tend to change their direction of flow. This is especially true of the Amu-Darja in the USSR, in its middle section and at its mouth.

The observed regularity and certain recurrence of floods makes it possible to predict and map them, and then to plan measures to prevent those of both natural and anthropogenic origin. Indispensable in this respect are thoroughly detailed analysis of the consequences of previous floods. Close study of the historical facts enables one to determine the character of damages and what is typical of floods in a particular region. Table 18 is a summary of the consequences of catastrophic floods which took place in the territory of what is today the USSR between 1824 and 1968.

Though far from being comprehensive, it illustrates the following points:

a) in particular territories, floods recur with a determinable frequency;
b) the scope of damages and injuries is considerable;
c) there has been an increase in both the frequency of floods in the USSR in the second half of this century and their consequences.

Part of the reason is the increase in population growth and density in the vulnerable territories and the construction of large industrial projects in these areas.

Extremely heavy damages are caused by flooding of the Brahmaputra, Ganges, Mekong, Mississippi, Missouri, Ohio, Po, Hwang Ho, Yangtze, and other rivers. The situation today is not better than it was in the past.

The Hwang Ho and Yangtze flood in 1887 caused the death of a million people; the Yangtze flood of 1931 took 140 000 lives, and altogether brought suffering to about 10 million people.

All the wealth and progress of the United States of America did not prevent the flood of the Ohio and Mississippi Rivers in 1937, which covered about 72 000 km^2, including the cities of Pittsburgh, Louisville, and Cincinnati. One and a half million people were made homeless [95]. Another catastrophic flood struck the state of Utah, badly damaging Salt Lake City, in June of 1983 (see Fig. 17, showing the city's flooded main streets). The energetic measures undertaken by the authorities limited the injurious effects and the gravity of the consequences. Sandbags were effectively used to artificially channel the water and mudflows. Some of the sacks were covered with plastic. As always in such cases, there was a shortage of materials, and the time for providing rescue was limited.

On the basis of my own observations, I recommend the quick assembling of protective barriers to direct flows where desired. These are portable and mounted on plastic constructions. Made of light synthetic materials, they can normally be used by municipal and other administrative organs of regions susceptible to floods as equipment for kindergartens, sports grounds, entertainment, and other public services.

Generally speaking, the readiness to organize efficient preventive and protective measures for the event of a flood can be characterized as very insufficient. As a result of the 1967 flood in northern India, which was caused by strong monsoon rains, 2 million people were made homeless in six states. Fifty million suffered from

Table 18. Summary of major floods in the USSR, 1824–1968

Location of flood (river, lake, or sea)	Date	Consequences
Neva	1824	In St. Petersburg, 324 houses destroyed, 3237 other constructions damaged; 208 died (official reports), 4000 (unofficial sources) [245]
Neva	1924	Leningrad region, Vasiliyevsky island, parts of central, Byborgsky, and Volodarsky regions flooded; port, number of plants and factories damaged [245]
Velikaya	1845	Town of Pskov badly damaged [95]
Dnieper	1845	Kiev and Kremenchug damaged [95]
Uzh	1810, 1833 1849, 1853	Town of Tula damaged [95]
Oka, Volga and Moskva	1908	50 000 left homeless [95]
Azov sea, southeast coast	1914	3000 died, town of Temriuk [166]
Azov sea, southeast coast	1969	Coastal settlements from Peresyp to Primorsk-Akhtarsk damaged [166]
Volga	1926	Kazan and other Volga towns damaged [194, 95]
Far East rivers	1927	Vladivostok (partially), Imai, Nikolsk-Ussurijsk, Ussuri Station covered with water [200]
Yenisei	1941	Krasnoyarsk damaged [95]
Severnaya Dvina	1946, 1947 1953, 1966	Arkhangelsk damaged [10, 190]
Dniester	1948, 1967 1969	Towns and villages of Moldavia damaged [32]
Zapadnaya Dvina	1956	Towns and villages of Belorussia, Latvia, Polotzk, Vitebsk, and others damaged and/or totally flooded [95]
Emba, Turgai, Tobol, Temir, Denkul, and Chagan	1957	Northwest Kazakhstan damaged [95]
Arys and Assa	1958	Southern and southeastern Kazakhstan damaged [95]
Lugan, Ol'khovaya, Severnij Donetz, and others	1964	Voroshilovgrad and administrative region damaged [32]
Lefu, Sujfun, Mo, Majkhe, Sintukhe, Monchukhai, Yanchikhe, and others	Aug./Sept. 1965 (twice)	Considerable part of Primorie area (including towns of Ussurijsk and Nakhodka) flooded and heavily damaged [Krasnoye Znamia, 1965, No. 200, 209]
Volkhov, Lovat, Sheloni, Msta, and Polisti, and Lake Ilmen	1966	Parts of Novgorod and Leningrad regions flooded [32]
Lower Danube	Jan./Feb. 1967	Town of Vilkovov (95%) flooded; Soviet river towns under threat of flood [205]
Kura and other rivers of Georgia	1968	Considerable part of Georgian republic damaged (esp. town of Borzhomi) [353]

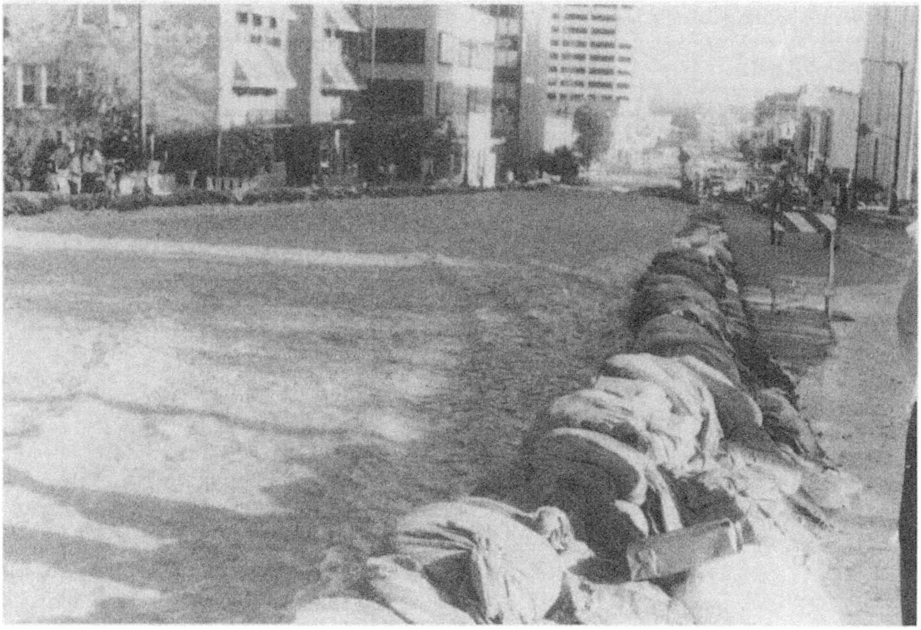

Fig. 17a–c. Central streets of Salt Lake City (USA) during the flood in June 1983 (Author's photo). **b, c** see p. 50

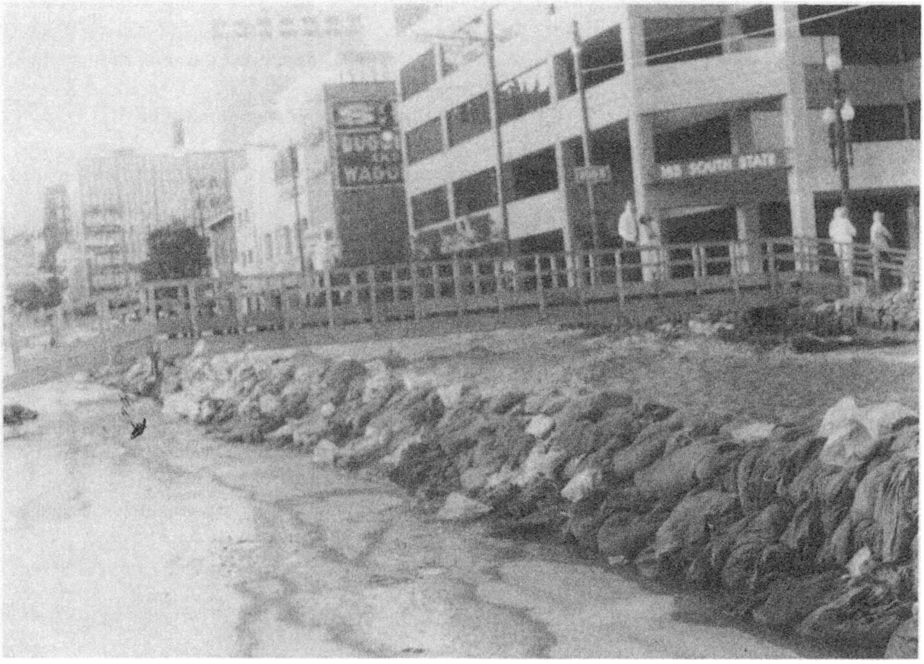

Fig. 17b

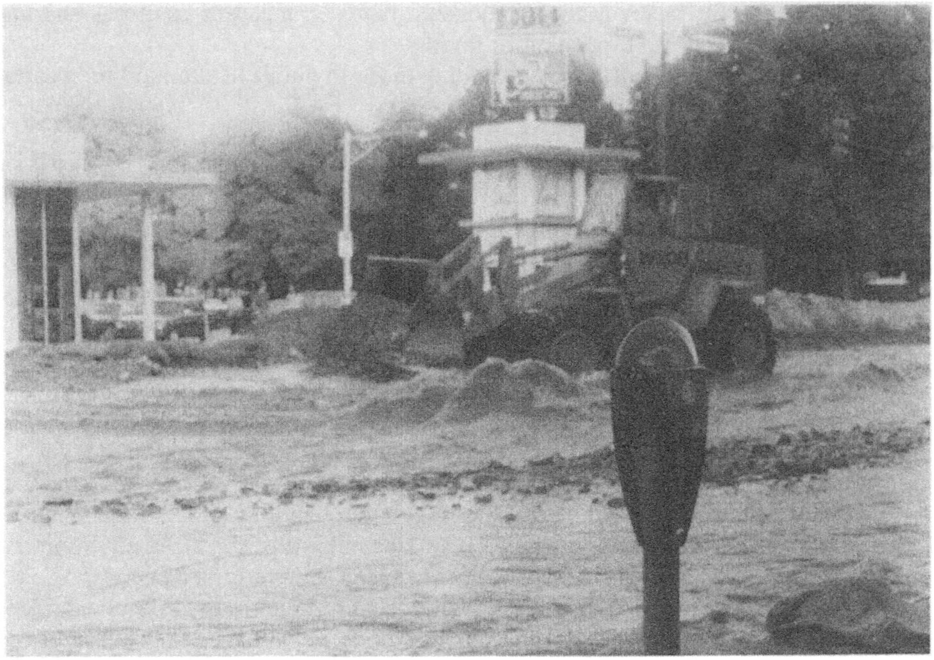

Fig. 17c

the flood which took place in the state of West Bengal in the first half of 1967 [299]. Eighty percent of Bangladesh was flooded in 1974; 2500 died, and about 37 million suffered from the disaster. Prior to this flood there had been five heavy ones in this area between 1962 and 1970.

These facts give us only part of the picture. Countries differ greatly with respect to their geographical conditions, level of industrial development, and economic and social arrangements. With respect to the implementation of measures for protection against floods, however, these differences are not considerable: Mass injuries always come suddenly, and the damage is always great. A sudden flood in January 1967 killed 1500 people in Rio de Janiero; 500 were made homeless. This flood was followed by another on February 20 of that year, which took 200 lives and rendered 25 000 homeless [300].

The main obstacles to the prevention of, and protection against floods are:

1. The absence of reliable, scientifically based forecasting, and the lack of foresight on the part of decision-makers
2. The shortage of material resources and trained personnel, and the lack of a functioning system of cooperation and coordination between organizations and institutions able to perform the complex and expensive activities required
3. Difficulties in overcoming phlegmatism, complacency, and a fatalistic attitude

Another important factor is the relationship between adjacent countries sharing the same geographical predisposition to floods.

The grave consequences of floods, including those to public health, and the deaths and drownings, are due to

a) the fast-flowing water;
b) damages and injuries caused by destroyed constructions, falling rocks, and landslides;
c) the hydrodynamic and hydrostatic effects of waves (in sudden floods);
d) unfavorable environmental conditions created by disturbances to the water supply (including water pollution), worsening of residential and domestic conditions, increased humidity, sudden cooling, and the stress on the population.

In Portugal in 1967, 450 people were killed in a flood. Lisbon was threatened with a lack of food and drinking water. In the town of Aminerom many people went without food, water, clothing, and medical aid [301]. There was a danger of epidemics. Strong, suddenly appearing floods bring about considerable deaths, injuries, and public health problems. On the other hand, slowly advancing, prolonged floods covering large territories cause greater disruption of the environment and appear more dangerous when considered from a long-term perspective.

The peculiarities of the public health and related conditions are studied here, using as examples for illustration catastrophic floods which have taken place in the USSR. In early 1964, the hydrometeorological service warned of a possible flood in the Voroshilovgrad region (Ukraine). The flood came in the second half of March. As a result of the overflowing of the Severny Donetz, Lugan, Krasnaya, Ol'khovaya, Derkul Belaya, and Aidar rivers and of reservoirs situated on the upper reaches of some rivers, the municipal districts of Artiomovsky, Kamenobrodsky, and Oktiabrsky were totally flooded, and the towns of Kremennoye, Lisichansk, Starobelsk, Svatovo, and others were partly flooded. In total, 11 244 houses, 26 kolkhozes and sovkhozes, and many industrial enterprises were flooded, and 23 409 people had to be evacuated. More than 35 150 people were involved in the construction of protective hydrotechnical structures and in rescue operations. There were a total of 58 559 people who needed medical and housing aid. The following health institutions were flooded as well: in Voroshilovgrad, Children's Hospital No. 4, Municipal Hospital No. 4, Children's Houses No. 1 and 3, the Children's Tuberculosis Sanatorium and the Crèche; in the town of Svatovo, the regional hospital and the maternity home. The pediatrics department of the Kremennoye Municipal Hospital and the hydropathy center in the town of Starobelskoye were threatened by the waters.

The Voroshilovgrad municipal sanitary-epidemiological station reported that the flood covered some pumping stations and sections of the water supply system (water wells nos. 1 a, 2, 3, and 4 of Lenin Square). The water became polluted, and the *Escherichia coli* titer showed the following indices: 6.0, 8.0, 10.0, 25.0, 91.0, 125.0, and 143.0. Of 490 bacteriological analyses of the water, 87 (17,7%) deviated from the norm, and of 500 chemical analyses, 25 (5%) did not meet the standards required by the Soviet standardization authorities [32, 34].

The situation just described can be observed in other cases as well; it is typical and recurrent. The North-West Board of the USSR hydrometeorological services an-

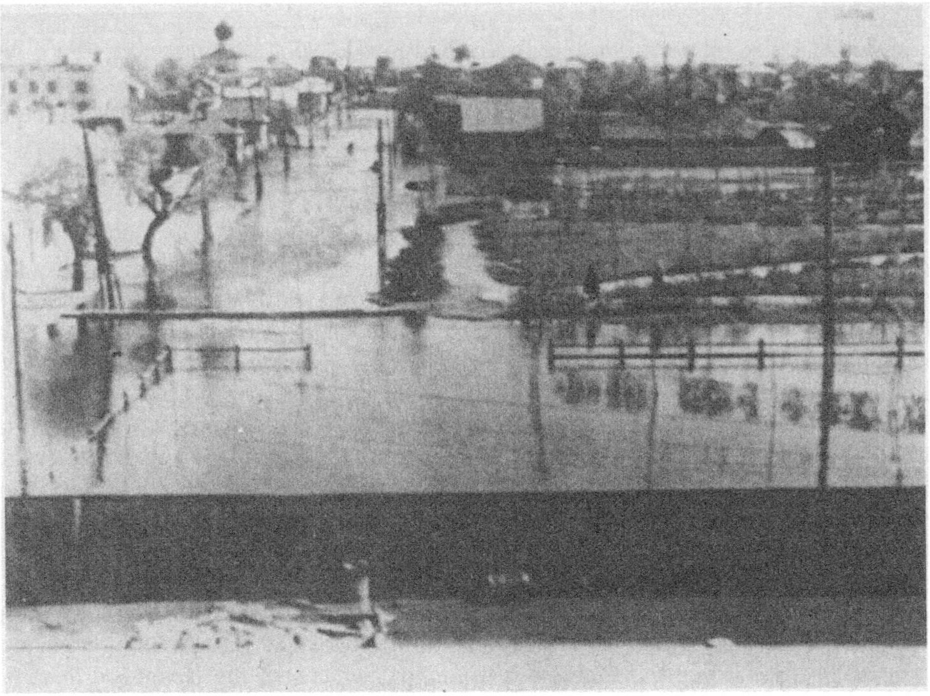

Fig. 18. View of the flooded part of the town of Staraya Russa [32]

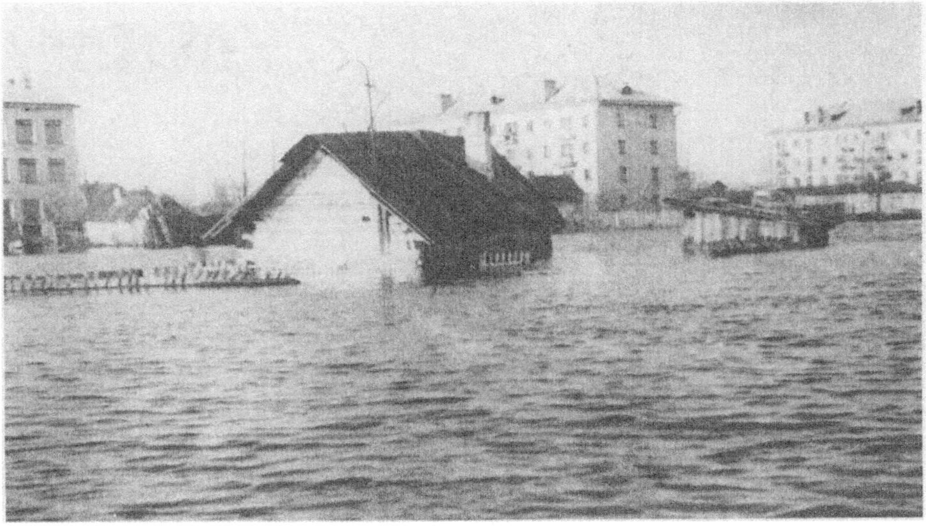

Fig. 19. A view of the flooded part of Novgorod [32]

nounced the possibility of flooding in the Novgorod region on March 12, 1966. As a result of heavy precipitation and unusual (for the first time in 40 years) spring freshets of the rivers Msta, Lovat, Polista, Shelon and Volkhov, and of Lake Ilmen, in the town of Staraya Russa, the Novgorod, Chudovo, and Malo-Vishersk districts were flooded (Fig. 18 and 19). In the town of Novgorod, the districts of Moshinsky, Selezky, and Lubitinsky were partially flooded.

The water began to rise on April 1, 1966, and reached its apogee on May 13, in Novgorod (at 765 cm above the ordinary level) and on May 12, in Staraya Russa (at 611 cm above the ordinary level). In the latter town, 41.3% of the streets were totally flooded, and 28.8% partially. The water began to fall on May 12, and continued to recede until the middle of July. The injurious consequences of the flood lasted for more than 2 months.

The flood badly affected 97 settlements, 92 collective farms, and the large workers' settlements of Proletarij and Krasnofarfornij. Four thousand houses were flooded, 540 km of roads destroyed, and 518 bridges and constructions for river crossing washed away. The following enterprises and institutions ceased to function: the Krasnij Farforist porcelain plant (Fig. 20), the knitted goods factory, the food works, the brick plant (Chudovo), municipal service institutions and industrial enterprises, public mess halls, stores, and other buildings (Staraya Russa). Many schools were closed. Among the health institutions damaged were the Staraya Russa municipal hospital and the sanitary-epidemiological station, the Novgorod hospital for infectious diseases, the Chudovo hospital, and the Krasnofarfornij hospital.

The flood was the cause of considerable difficulties in supplying the population with quality drinking water. In addition, the sewage system was disturbed; outhouses and dust-holes were destroyed. Of the 454 samples analyzed to determine the bacteriological characteristics of the water supply in Staraya Russa in 1966, 230 (50%) did not meet the official standards [34]. Of 33 samples taken from artesian wells, 21 (i.e., more than half) were also substandard. Water pollution peaked

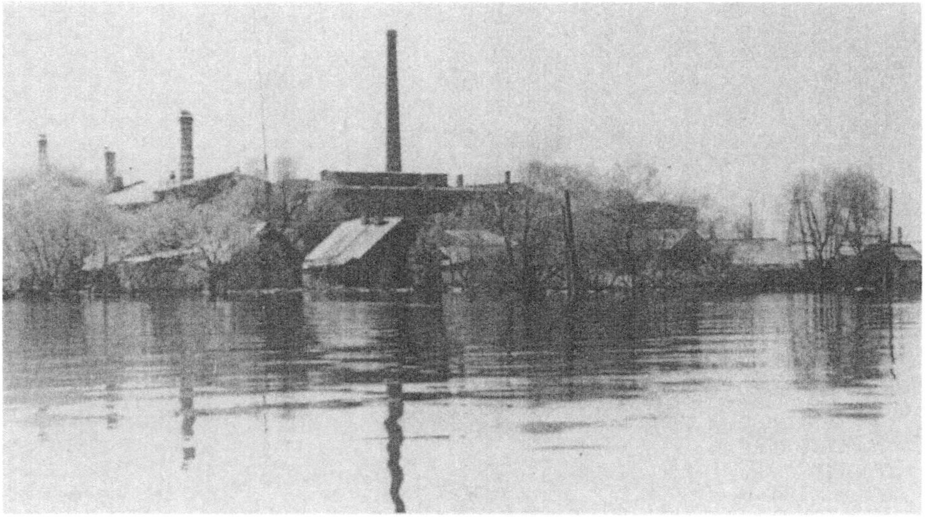

Fig. 20. Flooded porcelain plant, Krasnij Farforist, Novgorod [32]

during the period of the flood (April–June). The situation with the water supply system in the Msta branch of the Novgorod district was similar. Laboratory tests of samples from artesian wells showed a considerable increase in *E. coli* titer during the flood, which was a result of disturbances in the sewage system and general pollution in the territory. The quality of water taken from draw wells was also low. Testing of 68 such wells revealed an *E. coli* titer of no less than 300 in four of them, of 100 in 28 of them, and of 4.0 in 36.

Contamination of the water supply is a characteristic effect of floods. This can be illustrated with data reflecting the situation in Moldavia in 1969. As the water level of the Dniester rose, flooding its banks and covering drainage constructions, it became necessary to shut off the water supply to Kishinev through the main pipeline. According to a report from the Tiraspol sanitary-epidemiological station, the *E. coli* titer on June 18 was 37; on June 25, 56 [34].

Decreased water quality during floods predetermines an epidemiological chain reaction, where water is the chief medium for the spread of intestinal infections. The zoonotic disease leptospirosis (Germ. *Schlammfieber,* Eng. *swamp fever,* Fr. *fièvre des marais)* is transmitted mainly by polluted water. It was noted for the first time in Silesia in 1891, in connection with the Oder River flood. In 1926 the disease was reported in southern Bavaria, during the flooding of the Oder, the Elbe, and the Danube. Epidemics of this disease have been described in France, Italy, Japan, Australia, and elsewhere. As a preventive measure, it is advisable to organize a flood-warning system and to install drainage works in areas susceptible to the formation of stagnant water and bogs.

Table 19. Classification of floods

Origin	
Natural (unavoidable)	Predictable and avoidable by sanitation of the environment, supervision, control of construction, and proper use of hydroelectric structures
Appearance	
Sudden (within an hour): severe sanitary consequences and irreversible losses; among injuries, traumas and drownings prevail; time for organization and implementation of protective and rescue measures severly limited	Gradual (within days, weeks): severe sanitary consequences; diseases connected with unfavorable environmental conditions (colds, intestinal infections) prevail; generally, enough time for implementation of protective and rescue measures
Scope	
Limited (one or few settlements): some malfunction of municipal services; relatively minor damage to sanitary and residential constructions; mass evacuation	Large (number of regions, considerable part of the country): considerable damage to municipal, sanitary, and residential constructions; mass evacuation (tens, hundreds of thousands)
Duration of effects	
Short-term (1–2 days): unfavorable environmental effects minimal; rapid elimination of public health consequences	Long-term ($\geq$ 2 days, up to months): environment badly effected; liquidation of sanitary consequences takes much longer

Table 19 is a summary of the characteristics of floods, with regard to their origin, timing, territorial extent, duration of the ensuing calamity, and the public health consequences [34]. The classification demonstrates the necessity and the possibility of concrete planning for:

a) preventing floods and/or minimizing their effects;
b) protection from the effects of floods;
c) provision or medical aid to the injured and restoration of public health and safety.

Extensive research has shown that among the public health consequences of floods, traumas prevail. Most of these injuries are to the bones and joints of the extremities. During the 1966 flood in Staraya Russa, the water rose to the roofs of one-story buildings. Residents had to move in the streets by means of bridges specially built at the second-floor level. Health authorities reported ten times as many trauma cases there as in the previous year. In a dispensary in Voroshilovgrad, 62 trauma patients were treated in the second quarter of 1963, and 92 in the same period of 1964, representing an 80% increase [32]. The Bendery Republican Hospital (Moldavia, 1969) reported a 6.7% increase in these traumas over 1968. The Tiraspol hospital reported an increase of 11%.

Unfavorable environmental conditions during floods cause an increase in general morbidity. Table 20, based on data from a Voroshilovgrad dispensary, indicates an increase in

Table 20. Comparative incidence of some diseases reported by a Voroshilovgrad dispensary, 1963 and 1964 (the year of the flood)

Disease	Second quarter (n)		Increase (%)
	1963	1964	
Pneumonia (all forms)	4	17	320
Rheumatism	3	10	230
Stomach ulcer, duodenal ulcer	12	30	150
Gynecological diseases	8	12	50
Upper respiratory catarrh	199	284	40
Tonsillitis	47	62	30
Hypertension	40	60	50

Table 21. Morbidity in Staraya Russa, 1965 and 1966

Disease	Morbidity (‰)		Increase (%)
	1965	1966	
Tonsillitis	28.0	50.8	80
Upper respiratory catarrh	43.0	52.1	20
Lumbosacral neuralgia	30.0	41.8	40
Chronic otitis	6.6	11.1	70
Pneumonia	6.8	10.5	50

a) diseases where the factors of cooling of the environment and heightened humidity undoubtedly play a decisive role (respiratory catarrh, tonsilitis, rheumatism, pneumonia, gynecological disorders), and
b) chronic diseases exacerbated by environmental conditions, physical and psychological tension, disturbances in everyday life, and poor nutrition (hypertension, peptic ulcers).

Such was the health situation in the Novgorod region after the flood there. In Staraya Russa, which was in the flood zone, the general morbidity index increased by 41.7% between the years 1965 and 1966. Table 21 (based on data from the Staraya Russa municipal health service authorities [32]) gives a nosological breakdown of this increase.

As can be seen from the table, in Staraya Russa we have another example of the change in morbidity structure as a result of a flood; most particularly there is an increased incidence of those diseases most affected by rapid cooling of the environment and heightened humidity.

In Voroshilovgrad after the 1964 flood, and in Tiraspol in 1969 (after two successive floods) there was a marked increase in hypertensive disease, and in Tiraspol there was an increase in diabetes mellitus as well (Table 22; based on materials provided by the Tiraspol Republican Hospital [32]). These two increases are the effects of extended physical and psychological strain and trauma caused by the flood.

Grebeniuk et al. (in Mendelson [164]) report on the strong effect of flood conditions on blood pressure. During the Amur River flood of 1951–1952, a reading was taken of the entire population of one village struck by the flood (3600 people). Almost everyone showed a general increase in blood pressure. A similar testing was made of the population on the other bank of the river (which was not flooded), and only 20%–22% showed increased blood pressure.

Unfavorable environmental conditions badly affect children. Data on child morbidity in Voroshilovgrad (1964), as reported by the Municipal Children's Hospital No. 4, indicate that patients suffering from respiratory catarrh, tonsilitis, and pneumonia comprised 40.5% of the total. Considerable cooling and heightened humidity in residential buildings were most responsible for this. Measles and scarlet fever, i.e., infections which spread under worsened hygienic and domestic conditions, and because of forced closer contact between children, accounted for another 10.4% of patients. The overall situation hampered timely diagnosis, isolation, and hospitalization of patients, as well as thorough disinfection. The number of patients with these infections increased fourfold over the number for 1963.

Table 22. Incidence of hypertension and diabetes mellitus in Tiraspol, Moldavia, in 1968–1969 (per 10 000 population)

Disease	Total cases		New cases	
	1968	1969	1968	1969
Hypertension	101.0	107.3	7.2	10.0
Diabetes mellitus	44.8	51.5	4.8	7.6

The public health situation in Moldavia was similar after the flood of 1969. The health authorities of Rybnitzky district reported that, compared with the preceding year, the number of scarlet fever cases had doubled. In Tiraspol the number of such cases tripled, while there were twice as many cases of whooping cough. Increase in children's morbidity particularly is registered during the flood itself and in the period immediately following it (Fig. 21; based on data made available by the Staraya Russa municipal health authorities). The considerable increase in cases of whooping cough was observed during and after the flood, when a relatively large part of the town Staraya Russa was affected. The drastic cooling and high humidity caused a more severe course and frequent complications of the disease. There were 8.8 times more cases of whooping cough in Staraya Russa during and after the flood in 1966 than in 1965.

Floods cause the spread of other infectious diseases. According to Ryzhikov [211] and Sosnitzky and Nekrasova [239], they are responsible for the spread of tularemia in some regions of the northwest Russian Republic. A widespread outbreak of tropical yellow fever in Argentina in 1965–1966 was connected with floods that covered the area at that time (Olguin in [32]).

In discussing the public health consequences of floods, particular mention must be made of intestinal infectious. In Voroshilovgrad after the flood in 1954, typhoid and paratyphoid morbidity was almost twice as high as in 1953. A typhoid epidemic in Kishinev was directly connected with the June 1969 flood. Typhoid morbidity there was 9.8 per 100 000 in 1968, and 14.8 in 1969; this is an increase of 50%.

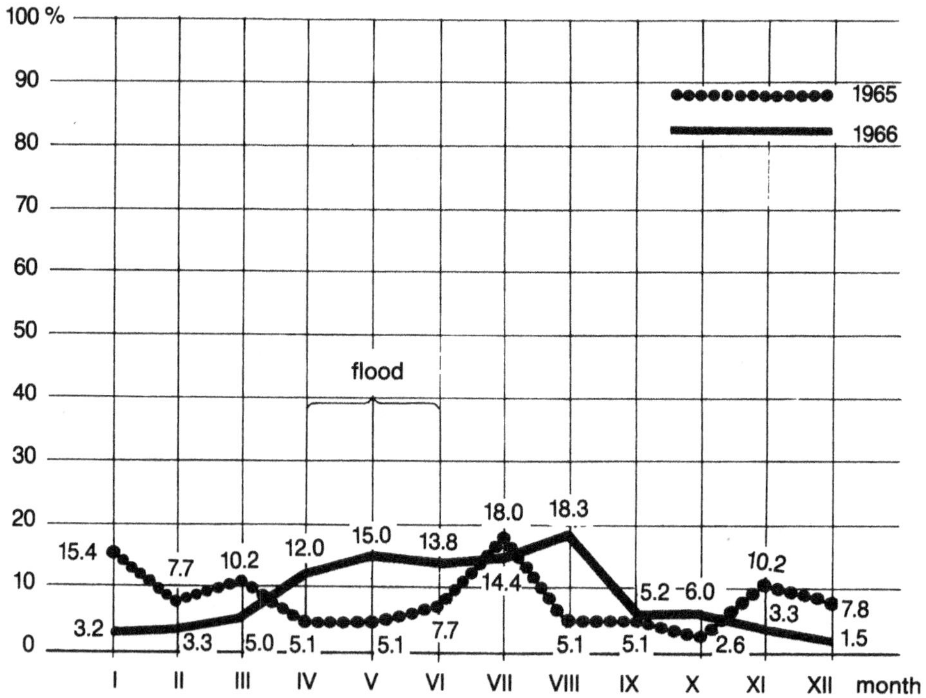

Fig. 21. Incidence of whooping cough in the town of Staraya Russa [32]

The 1966 flood in Novgorod brought about a drastic increase in dysentery – 400% over the preceding year in the Msta River area and 70% in the Novgorod district, which accounted for 33.5% of all cases registered throughout the Novgorod area. The cases of dysentery in Proletarij, the most damaged settlement along the Msta, accounted for 57.7% of all cases registered in this area. In the Chudovsky district the incidence of dysentery increased by 140% and in the town of Staraya Russa, by 240%. Among children the increase was especially great, in some places five times as much. The disease spread mainly through direct contact between the children. After the two successive floods in Moldavia in 1969; Tiraspol, Bendery, and Rybnitza were faced with an epidemic of dysentery [32].

Traumatic, somatic, and infectious morbidity increases are thus typical public health consequences of floods. Measures of prevention and provision of medical aid which can be implemented by the local public health services must be planned. Preplanning can have immediate positive results. For example, in early 1966 there was widespread dysentery in Krasnij Farforist (Novgorod region). Antiepidemic measures were implemented, which not only prevented the further spread of the disease during the flood, but even promoted its decrease, as is shown in Fig. 22 [32]. And in Rovigo, Italy, mass vaccination against typhoid and paratyphoid and improvement of the water supply system brought about a decrease in the incidence of disease. There were 5.8 cases of typhoid per 10 000 in 1956 and 4.2 per 10 000

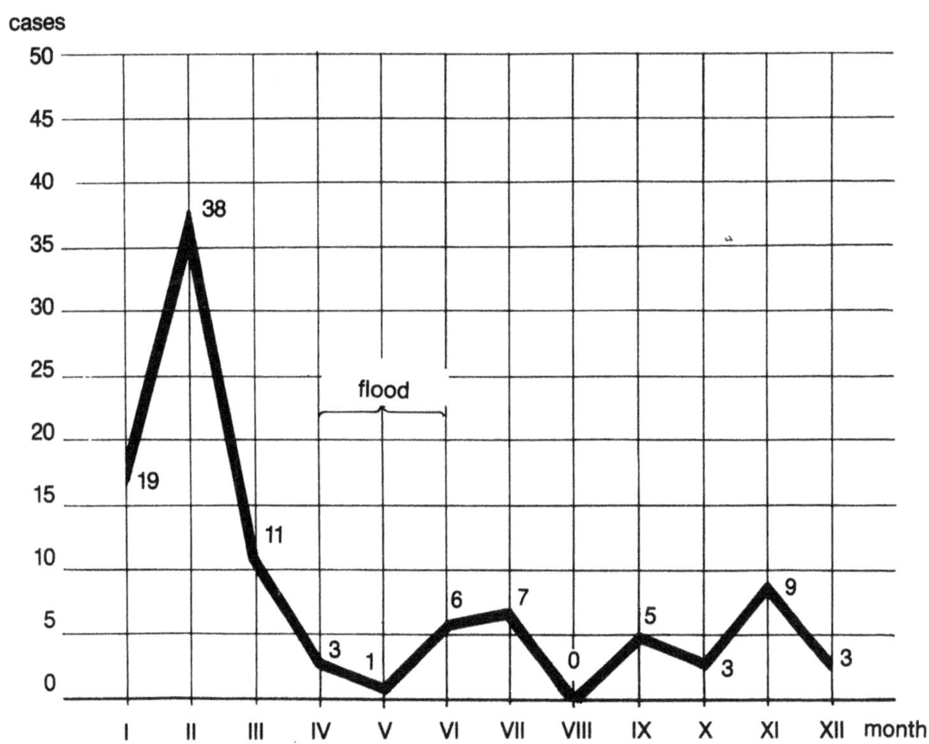

Fig. 22. Incidence of dysentery in the settlement of Krasnij Farforist, Novgorod region, (1966)

during the flood in 1965; there were 2.1 cases of paratyphoid per 10 000 in 1956 and none in 1965 [46]. Nonetheless, frequent floods in the southern part of the province prevented the health authorities from administering regular vaccination against diphtheria, and it has not been possible to eradicate this disease there.

Instead of passive fatalism, there should be active implementation of certain measures in communities or regions prone to flooding:

1. Natural and anthropogenic causes of floods at particular times and in particular areas must be considered
2. Industrial and agricultural development and the regulations covering culture and everyday life should be interconnected with a system of prevention and protection based on the potential damage that floods can cause
3. The state should supervise construction and operation of hydrotechnical plants, including protective dams, piers and reservoirs; it should supervise afforestation, and should provide for timely antiepidemic measures and medical aid in emergencies
4. There must be a sanitary and adequate water supply, both under normal conditions and in time of flood

Public Health Consequences of Mudflows and Snow Avalanches

Mudflows (torrents of mud and stones) and snow avalanches are considered together, with regard to their public health consequences and provision of medical aid to the injured, as natural disasters of mountainous regions and foothills. In the USSR these phenomena are frequent and their consequences grave. Their injurious effects are generally local. Their causes can be natural or anthropogenic, or a combination of both.

The danger lies in the fact that after such a flow or slide is triggered, the situation runs out of control. There are no efficient ways to predict such disasters, but their characteristic effects and, to a certain extent, the timing and location of their appearance are known to researchers. Thus, it is possible to organize, beforehand, a system of prevention and protection and provision of emergency aid to the stricken population.

Mudflows

Mudflows form in the beds of mountain rivers. They carry a high percentage of solid matter (10%–75%), which is the product of rock destruction. They can flow at speeds of 10 m/s or more [83].

The most common causes of mudflows are

a) heavy rains following prolonged precipitation which has already saturated the mudflow-forming rocks;
b) fast melting of mountain glaciers and snow as temperatures increase drastically;
c) seismic activity causing a rupture in a mountain lake or reservoir.

In Chile during a period of strong earthquakes, destruction of the El Cabra dam caused a mudflow which damaged part of the town. Eleven other dams were also damaged, though situated up to 100 km from the epicenter of the earthquake.

The descent of glaciers and falling rock crashing into mountain rivers can cause mudflows that then form large dams. When these burst, the mudflows cause further damage. On April 24, 1964, an avalanche weighing about 30 million tons crashed down the northern slope of the Zeravshanski mountain chain and blocked the Zeravshan River. Samarkand and its region, as well as other Uzbek and Tadzhik territories, were under the threat of flood.

Volcanic eruptions can also induce mudflows. This happened on the Kamchatka peninsula in 1956, when a large mudflow followed the eruption of the Bezymianij volcano.

Man's activities also cause mudflows, and this is of increasing concern in the USSR. Gussak and Besedin [112] have written about the effects of violation of topsoil vegetation and of improper exploitation of the soil on steep slopes. Disregard of regulations and laws relating to soil protection leads to erosion and, combined with uncontrolled felling of trees, this leads to mudflows. Reduction of the density of the forest means that a given territory is no longer provided with soil and water protection by the local flora [173].

Shipunov [226] notes that approximately one-third of the Lake Baikal waterbed and the adjacent territory has lost its natural water regulation capacity: the local landscape does not accumulate water and cannot distribute it evenly among rivers and springs. The author says that this situation, a result of man's activity, exerts a bad influence on the Pribaikal and Zabaikal landscapes. In the USSR, as in many other countries, the building of hydropower stations and reservoirs in the mountains has become widespread. Such a violation of nature brings about disturbances in the ecology. Miscalculations and errors made by designers can increase the possibility of ruptures in mountain lakes and reservoirs.

In the territory of Tajikistan alone, there are about 2800 blocked mountain lakes; this constitutes a potential threat of huge mudflows. In the past 100 years more than ten mountain lakes have broken their banks and caused catastrophic mudflows in the Central Asian republics [176]. Mudflows caused by ruptures of reservoirs and blocked up mountain lakes are distinguished by their enormous damaging power. An instructive example is the Issyk mudflow, which struck Alma-Ata on June 7, 1963. In the course of 6–7 h, several avalanches followed each other, and huge masses of water from Lake Issyk (2 km long, 600–800 m wide, up to 57 m deep) were displaced by mud and rock sediments [81].

Mudflows destroy communication lines, constructions, residential and public buildings, and health institutions. The flow I observed in September 1968 damaged public institutions in Yalta, including sanatoria. Gurzuf (Crimea) was especially hit, and there were human losses.

Five thousand mudflow beds have been registered in the USSR [54]. Their potential activity is a threat to towns and settlements in the foothill areas of the Transcaucasian republics (Azerbaijan, Armenia, Georgia), Kazakhstan and the Central Asian republics (Kirghizia, Tajikistan, Uzbekistan), the north Caucasus, Kamchatka, the Baikal region, and Sakhalin Island, and other areas in Russia, the Crimean peninsula, and the Carpathian region (Ukraine). Urban centers such as Alma-Ata, Dushanbe, Yerevan, Tbilisi, and Frunze are also endangered. Territories regarded as exposed to mudflows and avalanches within the USSR are shown in Fig. 23.

Other regions of the world vulnerable to mudflows are the mountainous areas of Bulgaria, India, Italy, China, the United States, Turkey, France, Yugoslavia, and Switzerland. The annual damage caused by mudflows in the USSR is estimated at 60–100 million rubles [81]. Table 23 shows the frequency of mudflows in the USSR and the damages caused by them.

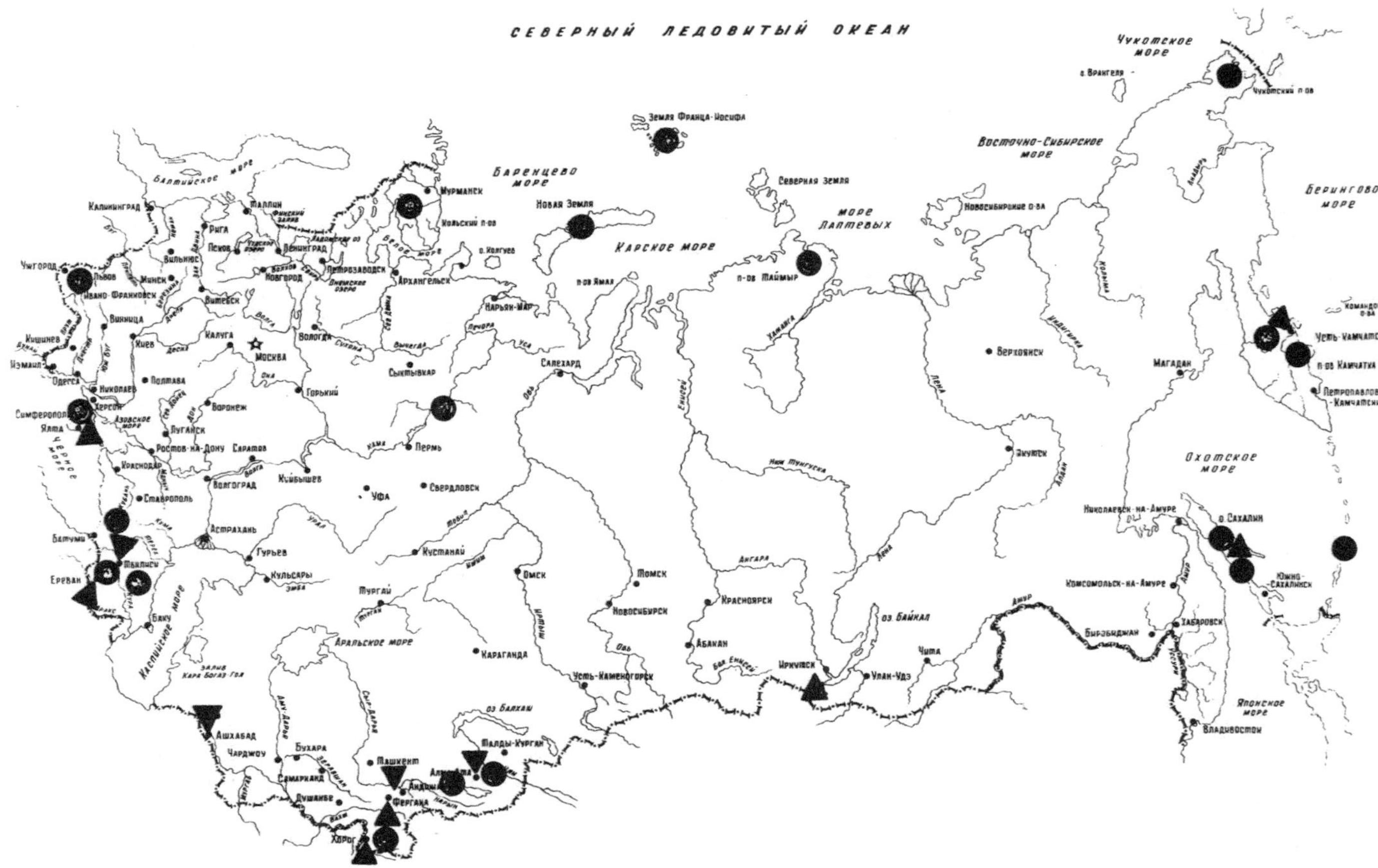

Fig. 23. USSR territories subject to mudflows and snow avalanches. ▲ Mudflows, ● Snow avalaches

Table 23. Mudflows in the USSR 1919–1967

Location	Date	Consequences
Shipchai river	1910	Total population of Bash-Geiinuk lost (400) [64]
Malaya Almaatinka riverbed	1921	Alma-Ata heavily damaged (500 lost) [68]
Shakhimardan river, Uzbekistan	1927	Part of Fergan town flooded, settlements of Shakhimardan and Vuazel flooded [64]
Getar river, Armenia	1946	1410 houses destroyed or damaged in Yerevan [64]
Issyk-Kul, mountains in the Zharsai ravine, Kazakhstan	1963	Residential buildings, bridges, other constructions washed away; people killed by 3 successive billows (Alma-Ata region) [64]
Isfairamsai riverbed, the mountain lake Yashinkul, Kirghizia	July 18, 1966	Dam crashed, result of billow attack 10–12 m high; flow carried woods, remnants of constructions; stormed approx. 7 h; many irrigational constructions, buildings, bridges, destroyed; power lines, gas mains washed away; many killed [243]
Chirchik, Angren, Naryn, and Kara-Darja (Uzbekistan)	1967	Andizhan, Tashkent, Fergana regions damaged, including Tashkent and Andizhan themselves; thousands of families evacuated [354]

The common effects of mudflows are large numbers of casualties within a short period of time; considerable destruction of residential, public, and other buildings, leading to unfavorable living conditions; and the need for mass evacuation from the disaster zone. The extent of the damage is determined by

a) the solid masses carried by the flux (stones, wood, remnants of destroyed buildings, etc.,) and its speed;
b) the hydrodynamic and hydrostatic effects of the mudflow waves; and
c) the fact that such a disaster occurs suddenly.

Muller (in Fleischman [81]) has written that the mudflow that started suddenly on October 9, 1963 in the Piave riverbed in northern Italy caused tremendous damage and took about 1900 lives. Fig. 24 shows the town of Langarone after it was destroyed by the resulting avalanche and landslide.

The situation is especially difficult and the consequences extremely damaging when the mudflow follows an earthquake. In Peru such a sequence of events took place on May 31, 1970. Underground tremors caused huge avalanches and snowslides in the ravines between steep snow-covered slopes of the Andes. The mountain lake Lianganuco flooded into the valley, bringing destruction to the towns of Yungai, Uaras, Caras, and Chimbote. More than 50 000 people were killed, and a million (of a population of 13 000 million) became homeless. The conditions in the mountainous regions were especially tragic, where the temperature fell to below 0° C [302]. This disaster and its grave consequences were the direct result of the combined effects of the earthquake and the mudflow and of the mountain conditions, with extreme environmental changes after the event.

The unfavorable environmental conditions caused by mudflows are similar to those caused by floods; thus, many aspects relating to these two phenomena are

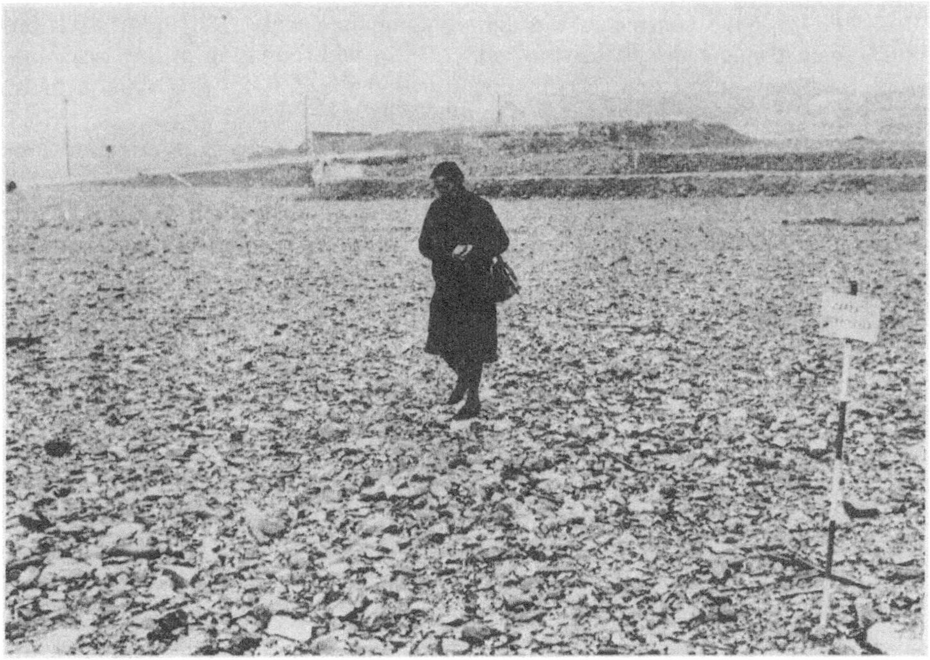

Fig. 24. View of the town of Langarone after it was destroyed by water avalanche and landslide (Nordisk, TASS)

identical. The prevalent injuries attributed to mudflows, especially in the initial period, are fractures of bones of the extremities, crush injuries, and multiple injuries to functionally important organs.

The mudflow which struck the Welsh village of Aberfan in 1966 killed 144 and injured 35. In 33% of cases, death was caused by asphyxia, in another 33% by crush injuries and multiple injuries to vitally important organs, and in the remainder by a combination of these effects.

The unfavorable environmental conditions caused by mudflows disturb normal living for a considerable period of time. Krayevaya [143] reported that the flow which appeared after the Bezymianij volcano erupted in Kamchatka in 1956 polluted the Kamchatka River, as a result of which the population of Ust-Kamchatsk was deprived of drinking water for 7 days.

The destruction of residential and public buildings, municipal institutions, and public utilities has serious consequences for public health, disrupting daily life. There is a great increase in intestinal infections, which are transmitted mainly through contaminated water. Rayushkin [206] notes that in Alma-Ata the typhoid morbidity index in 1950 was 49.2% of that registered in 1939, while following a mudflow in 1963 it was 70%, i.e., an increase of 40%. The source of the epidemic was mainly the bad water. The significance of water cannot be overestimated. For example, in Estonia in 1970–1975 impure water was the main agent that spread typhoid (55% of all registered cases [119]); of the registered cases of dysentery,

10.2%–49.7% were contracted through contaminated water. Of these infections, 58.6% were connected with private wells, 23.9% with pollution of the local water supply and sewage systems (by melting snow), and 12.1% with pollution of uncovered reservoirs [168].

As do floods, mudflows create new areal borders for carriers of infections, and water reservoirs become local sources of infection, especially in Central Asia.

The peculiarities of mudflows and their damages make them akin to another natural disaster, the snow avalanche. In many cases, their paths coincide. Both begin mostly on unwooded or felled mountain slopes [250]. This anthropogenic characteristic must be paid special attention.

Snow Avalanches

Two types of avalanches are generally distinguished, those consisting of friable, crumbly loose snow, and those consisting of solid, compacted snow. Low temperatures with strong winds combine to promote the formation of hard "snow planks"; in winter they are especially dangerous. The most damaging wet avalanches are those bearing soil, after a long thaw or heavy rains.

Avalanches are often triggered by drastic changes in weather conditions [79], such as a thick snowfall, rain-snow, fog, or a storm. Winter and spring torrents may also be dangerous. According to the US Ministry of Wood Husbandry [241], 80% of large snow avalanches start during or after heavy snowstorms.

Avalanches can also be caused by earthquakes (e.g., Chile, 1960; Alaska, 1964). The glacier movements in Tajikistan (1948) which caused avalanches were connected with the Khaitsk earthquake [65]. Avalanches may start on volcanic cones; this is relevant for the eastern regions of the Kamchatka and on the Kuril Islands. In 1959 and 1962, on Paramushir Island, avalanches started down the slopes of volcanic cones after several successive days of continous snowstorms. They covered houses and injured much of the population. The width of the avalanches reached 1000 m, while the height of the collapsed snowcap was no less than 20 m [304].

In the USSR snow avalanches are a serious problem. Up to 20% of the territory is vulnerable to them, including the mountainous southern belt of the country, beginning at the Carpathians and continuing up to the Sayans [251]. In several republics the danger is especially serious. In Kirghizia alone, 47.9% of the territory lies in the danger zone. Most active in this respect is the western Tien Shan. During the period 1950–1969, 3467 avalanches were registered here, with a total volume of 154.89 million m^3. Next in dregree of avalanche activity is the region of the inner Tien Shan [162]. Another dangerous region in the USSR is Sakhalin Island; avalanches here threaten such large settlements as Uglegorsk, Tomari, Chekhov, Kholmsk, Nevelsk, Bykov, and Sinegorsk. In one of the miners' villages, a powerful avalanche destroyed the houses and killed almost 100 people [123].

The USSR regions vulnerable to avalanches are the Khibinsk mountain chain, the Urals, Kamchatka, Chukotka, Taimyr, the Kuril and Komandor Islands (Russia); the Carpathians and the Crimean mountains (Ukraine); Pamirs, Tien Shan (the Central Asian republics); Zailijskoye Alatau (Kazakhstan); the Caucasus (Georgia)

[255] (Fig. 23). Snow avalanches also cause considerable damage in Austria, Italy, France, Switzerland, Yugoslavia, and Peru.

The damaging effects of snow avalanches are determined by

a) the accompanying airwaves and heavy snow pressure;
b) the traumatic effect of snow avalanches and of the rocks, wood, remnants of destroyed buildings, etc. they carry with them.

Table 24 indicates the possible extent of the consequences. An avalanche can leave a comparatively large number of casualties. The ratio of killed or lost to injured varies from 1:0.6 to 1:6.5. Men and children frequently prevail among the victims. Among the 14 buried under the snow in Austria in January 1951, six were men, three women, and five children [79]. In the Blons and Bartholomeber communities (Switzerland, 1954) children comprised 30.4% of those killed. At the sanatorium "Rock de Fiz" in the French Alps 79 people were killed in a snow avalanche in April 1970; 56 of them were children and 23 were staff. At the time of the catastrophe there were 185 children with tuberculosis in the sanatorium [305].

The fact that the victims are mostly men and children can be explained by the nature of the location where such disasters occur. More men engage in winter sports, while ill children are sent to health resorts in the mountains. According to the Austrian press, about 1000 people were lost in the Alps during one decade, 90% of them tourists [167].

Though the number of victims is considerable, it must be noted that the damages due to avalanches are not widespread. Groups of people are injured, and the tendency to greater population density in the mountains is increasing the danger of avalanches. In the USSR the number of people in mountainous areas, engaged in mining, hydroenergy construction, agriculture, and the rapidly developing tourism,

Table 24. Summary of major avalanches, 1910–1970

Location and date	Consequences	Ratio of killed/ lost to injured
State of Washington (USA), 1910	>100 killed when three trains crashed into canyon [32]	–
Swiss Alps, winter 1950–1951	234 buried in snow, 98 killed, 62 injured [79]	1:0.6
Italian Alps, 1951	46 killed [79]	–
Austrian Alps, 1950–1951	135 killed, 188 injured [79]	1:1.4
Yugoslavia, 1951	25–30 killed [79]	–
Blons and Bartholomeber communitites (Switzerland), 1954	102 killed, including 31 children; 250 made homeless [79]	–
Santa Valley, Huascarán avalanche (Peru), 1962	6 settlements totally destroyed, 3 others partially destroyed; approx. 4000 killed [20]	–
Val d'Isère (France), 1970	48 killed, 60 injured [238]	1:1.2
Amoz-Koraz Valley (Turkey), 1970	31 killed, >200 injured [238]	1:6.5
Canton Valais (Switzerland), 1970	48 buried by avalanche, 18 rescued [238]	–

is constantly increasing. The situation is similar in other countries. In Tirol (the Austrian Alps) the population density in the valleys in 1961 was 260/km^2; a 50% increase is predicted by the year 2000 [160].

Avalanches lead to unfavorable environmental conditions, and can cause or contribute to combined injuries of the extremities and the thorax, frostbite, asphyxia, and respiratory diseases connected with overcooling. Mortality is extremely high under these circumstances. In France between 1965 and 1972, 117 people died in snow avalanches. The main causes of death were asphyxia caused by crushing of the thorax (84%); asphyxia caused by blockage of the respiratory tract (4%); overcooling (8%); trauma (4%) [74].

Two hours is the maximum time a person covered by a snow avalanche can stay alive. However, it is possible to survive beyond this limit, if one finds oneself in an air cavity under the snow. Flaig [79] describes a case of a man who was rescued from under an avalanche 13 days after he was buried by it; he was alive, but both legs had to be amputated. In general, depending on local conditions, rescue operations must be continued for at least 24 h [241].

Destruction of residential buildings, sanatoriums, and public institutions by snow avalanches badly affects living conditions, and extreme geographical conditions

Table 25. Comparison of mudflows and snow avalanches

	Mudflows	Snow avalanches
Location	Mountainous and foothill regions	Mountainous and foothill regions; vulnerable to landslides
Origin	Natural Anthropogenic	Natural Anthropogenic
Distribution of effects	Mainly local	Local
Reasons for appearance	Prolonged, torrential rain. Fast melting of snow and ice. Active seismic movement. Technological errors. Ecological disturbance of environment	Abundant snowfall, rain, and strong winds. High seismic activity. Ecological disturbance of environment
Factors causing damage	Large pieces of debris in flow. Hydrodynamic and hydrostatic effect of waves. Extreme character of mountain conditions	Accompanying areal wave. Traumatic injuries. People buried by snow. Overcooling
Public health effects	Injuries, drownings. General morbidity increase, esp. intestinal, infectious, and respiratory diseases	Injuries, asphyxia. Frostbite. Increase in respiratory diseases
Preventive and rescue aid	Complex agroengineering activities. Mudflow prediction service. Mobile teams for rescue and medical aid	Afforestation and other agroengineering activities. Mobile teams for rescue and medical aid
Time of implementation	Ongoing, constant agroengineering activities rescue and medical aid from moment of appearance	

exert an unfavorable influence on rescue operations. All this is quite common in the USSR. A few days after the sanatorium "Sakhalin" (in the Sakhalin region) was opened in January 1965, its main residence was hit by an avalanche of dry snow, which had a volume of 8500 m^3. It destroyed the medical treatment department and the bedroom wings. The cost of antiavalanche protection for the sanatorium complex was 310 000 rubles [123].

In the spring of 1966 a massive avalanche descending into the valley of the Bolshaya Almaatinka River (Kazakhstan) disturbed the functioning of the municipal water supply system. Communication and electrical lines were damaged. The highway leading to Alma-Ata was closed to traffic for 12 days [306]. This situation badly hindered rescue operations and provision of emergency medical aid.

It is evident that here, as with mudflows, prescience is needed. Table 25 characterizes the differences between mudflows and avalanches, and suggests an orientation for concrete, purposefully planned activities, such as:

1. Forecasting and mapping, taking into consideration the interconnected and interdependent anthropogenic and natural causes
2. Sanitation of the environment in mountain and foothill seismoactive areas susceptible to mudflows and avalanches
3. Readiness to maintain and respond to an information service with personnel and equipment and the capacity to provide emergency medical aid to the injured

The range of the public health services' participation in these activities must be as wide and comprehensive as possible. In practice this means antiavalanche and antimudflow measures, forest protection, engineering and construction development to solve the ecological problems relevant to mountain and foothill areas. As experience has shown, it is imperative to prevent further uncontrolled urbanization of these areas.

Public Health Consequences of Mass Hunger

Famine as a natural disaster is determined by a combination of natural and social factors. Two aspects are relevant to the problem of malnutrition, the biomedical and the sociocultural. Among the natural causes are failed harvests and droughts resulting from meteorological conditions [17]. Hunger follows where crops have been destroyed by floods, typhoons, or such biological phenomena as swarms of locusts. Hunger can also be a consequence of volcanic eruptions. The one on Iceland on July 20, 1783 killed 75% of the cattle within 40 days. This was due to poisoning by fluorine and other elements and compounds from the lava flow, and to the lack of grass, which had been burnt under the volcanic ash. One-fifth of the total population (i.e., 100 000 people) died of hunger and disease [271].

Special attention must be paid to failed harvests caused by ecological disturbances and poor agricultural management. Of particular concern here is exaggerated monocultural specialization (sugar cane, coffee, rubber-yielding plants, etc.). There is also a lag of agricultural production behind population growth in many parts of the world (China, India, Egypt, Jordan, etc.). In combination with social and economic problems, this lag leads to mass hunger.

The Western industrial countries contain 20% of the world's population and produce about one-third of the world's grain, while the developing countries contain 50% of the world's population and produce not even one-third. The figures are even more striking for meat and dairy products: 30% of the world's population produces 70%–80% of the goods [237].

More than half of the world's 3.7 billion people are starving [44]; only 1.3 billion are adequately nourished. The situation does not appear hopeless, as the limits of agricultural production have not yet been reached. The high productivity of such countries as the United States, Canada, Australia, France, and Israel offers encouraging proof of this. It is not by chance that 50% of the world's grain exports come from the United States and the other 50% from Canada, Australia, France, and Argentina [26].

China has long been referred to, as the land of hunger. Research undertaken by Nanking University cites 1829 occasions of hunger, frequently on a mass scale, in China in the course of the past 2000 years [51]. In 1877–1878 a famine took the lives of 9–13 million people [183].

In the Middle Ages, Europe was striken by famine every 8–10 years. In 1847, in Ireland alone, a million people starved to death. The situation has not changed for the better in the present century. The widespread hunger in the USSR in 1921–1922 as a result of drought and poor harvests affected a huge portion of the population. Data relevant for January 1, 1921 indicate that approximately 15 million people were starving; by July 1922 this number had risen to 22 million [105].

Droughts and the hunger they cause affect many countries on a mass scale, even today. In the middle of 1973 a drought laid waste to a vast area of West Africa, 4000 km long and 1000 km wide, encompassing Chad, Mali, Mauritania, Niger, Senegal, and Upper Volta; six million people were threatened with death [63].

History provides many examples of two disasters following each other: drought and flood. In China, 3106 floods and 1873 droughts followed by widespread famine were registered between 206 B.C. and 1911.

Frequently, mountain landslides (triggered by earthquakes), floods, collapsed mines, communication failures, and shipwrecks cause hunger of a local character, affecting individuals or small groups of people.

One of the grave results of natural disasters is infant malnutrition because of disturbances in the production of breast milk. This was the case after the Guatemalan earthquake of February 4, 1976; nutrition was not a great problem in general, because the disaster occured during the harvest period [270].

The ever increasing danger of famine has become one of the most pressing problems facing mankind. In the 1960s, 10%–15% of the world's population was suffering from hunger; when those receiving inadequate nutrition were added, the figure rose to 50% [177]. The long-term perspective is not encouraging. The natural capacity of the environment for self-regulation is gradually being undermined by man's activities. Hunger is expected to increase, particularly in the developing countries. At the Second World Food Congress in the or The Hague in 1970, it was reported that hunger and malnutrition are the constant lot of one billion people [136]. Some believe that by the year 2000 the mortality due to hunger may double [165].

The main reasons for hunger are

a) the social and economic disorder in the modern world, the confrontation of different political regimes, ideologies, cultures, and
b) anthropogenic ecological problems, the energy crisis, and the population explosion.

Parrack [192] connects the problem of hunger with the successive appearance of complex predisposing and "triggering" factors. Famine itself is often preceded by a prolonged period of insufficient nutrition. Limitations in the ecosystem itself cause resources such as the soil to become periodically exhausted, and under conditions of annual drought, strong hurricanes, floods, military actions, etc., hunger follows. Social causes of significance include all types of war, which frequently invoice blockades of cities or settlements. Wars ruin a country's economy and impair the population's health. Three of the horsemen of the Apocalypse – war, famine, and pestilence – ride together in this situation [109].

Extreme ideological and political trends bring about changes of political power, and are frequently accompanied by drastic social and economic reforms which can also lead to mass hunger. Illustrative examples are the industrial revolution in Britain (late eighteenth to early nineteenth centuries) and the collectivization of

Table 26. Causes and effects of famine

Causes	
Natural:	Social:
Drought	Wars, including civil wars and blockades
Crop destruction by floods, typhoons, or other natural disasters, including biological ones, such as crop devastation by locusts	Crisis and destruction of the economy due to war or socioeconomic disorder
Catastrophes (crashes of mountain rocks, mines); communication malfunctions, shipwrecks, etc.	Essential socioeconomic reforms lacking in the country
Disasters of anthropogenic origin (ecological disturbances, energy crisis, bad management causing agricultural output to fall behind the demands of growing population)	Free will, as means of expressing protest or struggle for human rights or other goals
Territorial extension	
Local: population involved can be strictly limited or vast masses	Great: usually involving vast masses of people
Movement of population	
Mass migration: escape, evacuation, emigration	Natural population movement: increase in mortality, decrease in birth rate
Morbidity increase	
Respiratory diseases, tuberculosis, metabolism disturbances	
Psychological disturbances	
Infections: parasitic typhus (epidemic typhus, relapsing fever), intestinal and children's infections	
Poisoning (food, ergotism)	

agriculture and industrial management reforms in the USSR in the 1930s. Hunger-strikes by particular groups and individuals are a means of protest in the struggle for human rights or other goals. Table 26 summarizes the sociohygienic characteristics of hunger and its causes, extent, and consequences.

In spite of the relative remoteness of events, it is instructive to consider the reliably documented data on the widespread hunger in the USSR in 1921–1922 and in besieged Leningrad in 1941–1942. The first of these famines involved a tremendous area including the Urals and the Ukraine, and was caused by a severe drought in the Volga region. But it was not only the drought; other factors, mostly social, also affected the situation. In fact, it was a unique combination of sociopolitical, economic, and military developments, which brought about:

1. Disintegration of the economy and destruction of industry and the transportation system (the direct results of 7 years of war – the First World War, 1914–1918, and the civil war of 1918–1921
2. Radical social, political, and economic reforms connected with the October Revolution (1917), which created the lack of materials and of experienced professionals
3. International isolation of the USSR

All this directly affected the public health situation. After the grave consequences of two wars, mass migrations, and epidemics, a functioning system of public health services no longer existed. A large part of the population was entirely without qualified medical help, and there were no agents or means found to work toward eliminating the hunger and its consequences.

Malnutrition had been observed in several parts of the Soviet Union prior to the famine of 1921–1922. The newspaper *Severnaya Kommuna* reported on the daily bread ration in Petrograd in November 1918: 200 g for the first category; 100 g, 50 g, and 25 g for the second, third, and fourth categories of the population. Gorky wrote: "Those who suffered most of all were the children, then people engaged in intellectual activities, those working in offices and laboratories, since they were not adaptable enough to practical life and had no experience in the cruel struggle for a piece of bread" [257].

The following data provide a general idea of the extent and character of the hunger [307, pp. 1–4]. The 1920 census registered 1 258 132 residents in Bashkiria; 90% of them suffered from hunger. In Tataria, with a population of 2 852 135, of which 1 304 420 (45.7%) were children; 1 698 054 people (59.5% of total population) of which 740 843 were children (56.7% of total children) were starving. Of the 1 316 980 people in Cheliabinsk, 780 950 were suffering from hunger (59.2%) [308, pp. 14–17]. These figures are evidence of the mass scale of the disaster.

In the course of time, in some places such as the Volga region, the situation became so desperate that orache, clay, and bark were used as food, and old sheepkins were cooked and eaten [307, p. 2]. This was the struggle for survival.

Man's capacity for fasting is assumed to be limited to 65–70 days. At Minnesota State University in 1940 a group of volunteers were maintained on a daily half-starvation ration of 1600 calories for 168 days [122]. Of course, a voluntary experimental situation cannot be compared to a true disaster, in which there is an atmosphere of helplessness and inconsolability in the face of suffering, especially of children.

Hunger causes various socially dangerous phenomena, such as delinquency, a decrease in the general cultural level, moral degradation, and hunger psychoses (cannibalism) [185]. Reports from regions that were badly stricken by hunger in 1921–1922 give horrible examples of this. In the Ufa region, there were murders, mob rule, and cannibalism [307, p. 16]. In one family the mother was ill, and the children had been tied in different corners, for they were gnawing at each other. Another report [309, p. 39] stated that the mother of a starving family of seven, after 3 days of total hunger, cooked her deceased 1-year-old daughter to feed the children and herself (Feb. 1921). (The neighbors were told that the infant had been taken away to an orphan asylum). Such horrible occurrences are certainly isolated, but they cannot be ignored.

In extreme situations hunger leads to mass morbidity and mass mortality. In Tataria, 209 783 were registered as diseased, and the number of deaths caused by hunger reached 15 493 [308, pp. 14–17]. The abnormal domestic and sanitary conditions bring about a drastic increase in infectious diseases. Reports from the Kazan medical institutions give the following figures with respect to intestinal infections: dysentery, 18.6% of cases, mortality 74.6%; enteritis and gastritis, 13.4% of cases, mortality 18.6%; typhoid, 5.4% of cases, mortality 74.6% [308, p. 5].

The main reason for this increase in infectious diseases was the protein-caloric malnutrition, which seriously impaired the immune system of the body. It is generally known that there is a synergism between infections and malnutrition; infections and parasitic diseases are the main reason for protein-caloric insufficiency [161].

Fast, efficient provision of food directly to the starving population would certainly have improved the situation. But as that was impossible, the problem became one of mass evacuation. In Tataria it was necessary to evacuate 138 592 people [308, pp. 14–17]. The destruction of the transportation network, and the social and political disorder hindered implementation of appropriate evacuation measures. In chaos, refugees began to flee the territories stricken with hunger, and this stream of desperate people merged with the mass migration of war refugees (1914–1918 and 1918–1921). The Varshavsky evacuee distribution point at Petrograd reported that, in September 1921, refugees who had left the territories where there was great hunger comprised 57.5% of the total number transferred through this point [310, p. 61].

Toward winter, the migration of refugees by rail increased. In December 1921 in Petrograd alone, their number reached 30 000 from the Volga area; one-third of these were children [311, p. 21]. Under these chaotic conditions, parasitic typhus was spread rapidly by the newly infected. The combination of widespread hunger, disease, and mass migration led to pandemics of relapsing fever and epidemic typhus throughout the entire Soviet Union. In all, about 25 million people suffered from epidemic typhus, and 8–9 million had relapsing fever [247].

According to Gran and Matulsky [106], parasite-borne typhus of various kinds infected 20% of the population of the Ukraine, though they note that the actual morbidity was 4.2 times higher than that reported in official statistics. In four Jewish colonies, 72.8% of families had epidemic typhus and relapsing fever. Undoubtedly, the wave of Jewish pogroms in the Ukraine at that time played a considerable role here.

Hunger is a factor weakening overall resistance, and in combination with abnormal domestic conditions, excessive physical and neuropsychological stress, and the effects of overexposure, promoted increased morbidity and mortality, particularly among refugees. By September 26, 1922, among the refugees treated at hospitals in Petrograd there were 12 432 adults and 1099 children; of these, 2852 adults (22.9%) and 831 children (75.6%) died [312]. By October 1922 there were approximately 20 000 refugees in Petrograd. Comparative figures for Petrograd residents and refugees show that per 10 000 of the indigenous population, 6.6 cases of parasite-borne typhus were registered; for refugees this index was 175.5, i.e., 26 times higher.

The civil war and the pogroms made the consequences of hunger especially tragic for the Ukrainian Jews. In 1920–1922 the birth rate there, as compared with that for the prewar period, fell from 42.5 to 26 per 1000. In some Jewish colonies 20% of the population died of starvation. Mortality per 1000 was 40.5 in the Odessa region and 80.2 in the Yekaterinoslav region [106].

These facts reflect the medical consequences of the 1921–1922 famine in the Soviet Union. They are illustrative of a certain pattern to be observed under conditions of widespread hunger caused by droughts, and against a background of socioeconomic and political crisis. Any country is vulnerable to such a tragedy.

Mass hunger can also be accompanied by food poisoning, such as ergotism. In 1978, Pokrovsky and Tutelian [198] noted 150 cases of chronic ergotism in one African area; one-third of these patients died. Droughts and failed harvests in the previous 3 years had led people to eat bad-quality grain. Of 140 hospitalized, 47 died; the others needed amputation of their extremities. Destruction of the diseased grain stopped the morbidity.

Among the medical effects of hunger, then, we must consider:

1. Two successive stages: malnutrition and starvation
2. Problems of mass evacuation, or if that is impossible, of mass migration of refugees, due to the lack of appropriate aid
3. The aggravating effects of excessive neuropsychological and physical stress, and of overexposure to cold, or under certain circumstances heat
4. An increase in general and infectious morbidity and mortality, aggravated by the mass migration

In the USSR and elsewhere there are periodic droughts [313]. Certain features of these droughts enable scientists to predict their appearance. Although it is known that socioeconomic problems can lead to famine, the reverse is also true: widespread hunger may bring about socioeconomic and political crisis. Ethiopia is an example of this. A drought in 1973 led to a famine and hundreds of thousands of Ethiopians died. This disaster was followed by political and military events that are well known. What is not so well known is the gravity of the purely medical consequences of the famine. One of these is the weakening of the following generation. This can be prevented only by the timely provision of medical and other aid to the suffering population. A model for this is provided by documents on the 1921–1922 famine in the Soviet Union.

Also instructive are the data on the famine during the siege of Leningrad in 1941–1942. Though geographically confined to the city limits, the disaster took on a mass character in terms of the population involved. The famine was directly due to the blockade of the city by German troops, which began on September 8, 1941, and to the destruction of all food stores and warehouses by the German aerial bombardment. The civilian population found itself in direct confrontation with the army. As of September 2, the official ration had been decreased four times, and on November 20 the fifth ration-statement issued by the authorities during this short period of time announced that 250 g of bread was henceforth alloted to workers daily, and 125 g to office employees, dependants, and children [314].

On January 24, 1942 the water supply system ceased to function [315]. Hunger struck the city. Men suffered most of all, for they carried the main burden of physical labor, psychic trauma, cold, and hunger, which caused the high morbidity and mortality among them (Fig. 25). Mortality among women took on mass proportions 2–3 month later [91].

The Leningrad therapists Chernorutzky, Tushinsky, Gelshtein, Tur, and colleagues established the term 'alimentary dystrophy' to signify the disease caused by malnutrition and starvation. Early complications included bronchitis and pneumonia, as it was the cold season; these accounted for about 90% of the cases treated [92]. Complications related to damage of the gastrointestinal tract developed

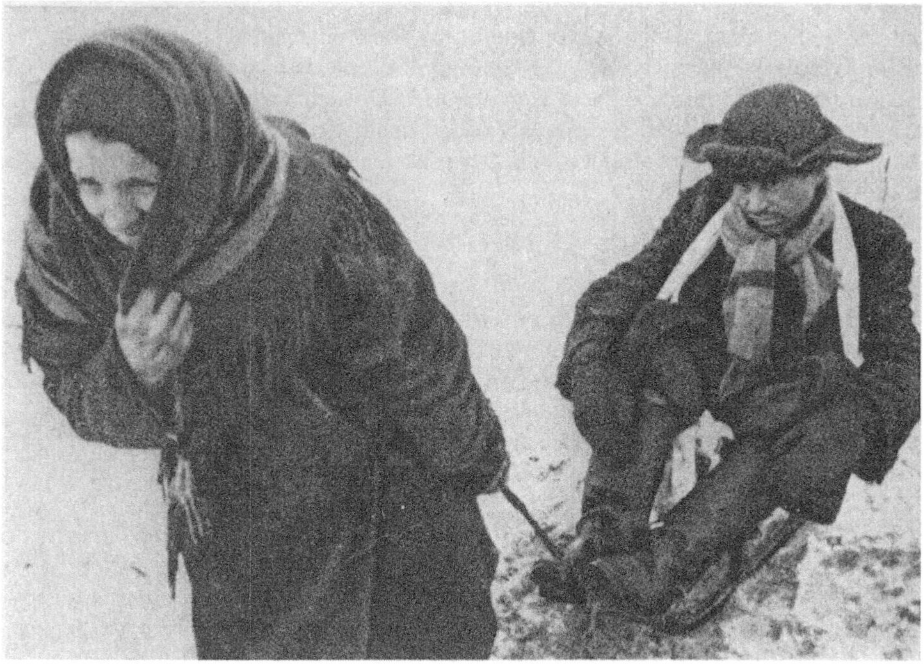

Fig. 25. A woman draws a starvation-weakened man on a child's sled [350]

next, followed by the spread of dysentery, typhoid, and epidemic typhus [49]. Then came scurvy, from which many died [316].

Beginning in the spring of 1942 there was an increase in cases of tuberculosis. Tushinsky was extremely concerned about this increase among children. According to Volovik's data [317], three-fourths of the children with tuberculosis died. The majority of lethal tuberculosis cases were registered for the first half of 1942. Shenderovsky (cited in [11]) adds that 83% of the Leningrad tuberculosis patients suffered from alimentary emaciation (inanition) [11].

The unusually severe and persistent psychic stress, coupled with heavy physical tension, created a peculiar clinical picture, as can be seen in the course and distribution of hypertensive diseases in Leningrad [149]. The percentage of those with hypertensive diseases as a proportion of those treated in the First Leningrad Pavlov Medical Institute increased from 3.7 in the prewar period to 27.5 by April 1943 [149].

The grave conditions of siege in Leningrad and the consequent hunger brought about a drastic increase in psychiatric illness as well. Before the war, in 1940, 1.1 per 1000 people were psychiatric patients; by the second quarter of 1942 this figure had reached 4.8 [318]. Psychoses caused by alimentary dystrophy were particularly severe, and more than 50% of such cases ended in death [249].

Table 27. Births and deaths as proportion of total population in Moscow and Leningrad, 1940–1944 (‰)

	1940		1941		1942		1943		1944	
	Births	Deaths	Births	Deaths	Births	Deaths	Births	Deaths	Births	Deaths
Moscow [319]	25.3	15.6	22.9	18.8	12.7	27.6	8.5	21.8	17.1	19.9
Leningrad [320]	22.0	17.6	25.4	42.4	9.7	360.0	12.6	40.3	30.4	16.8

Morbidity and mortality due to hunger affect the natural growth of population. Table 27 illustrates this point using the case of besieged Leningrad, and comparing the birth and death rates in Moscow and Leningrad for 1940–1944. Military activities must also be taken into consideration here.

The table shows a decrease in the birth rate and an increase in mortality during the war, the most extreme period being late 1941 and early 1942. The birth rate in Moscow in 1942 was half that of 1940, while mortality had increased 1.8 times. In Leningrad the corresponding figures were a factor of 2.3 for the birth rate decrease and of 20.4 for the increase in mortality. The blockade and famine were clearly responsible for this. Within a relatively short period (late 1941 to mid 1942) three-quarters of a million people died in Leningrad [321]. According to unofficial data, during the entire period of blockade more than one million died.

Among the problems facing the health authorities in Leningrad, hunger was of the utmost importance. It caused many deaths directly, increased the general and infectious morbidity, and exacerbated the extremely difficult conditions under which the health services were working.

The health service personnel itself was starkly reduced due to illness and death. In a letter from Dr. Nikitsky, head of the municipal health department, to Popkov, chairman of the Leningrad municipal soviet, Nikitsky states that on October 10, 1941 there were 41 physicians responsible for 800 beds in the "25th of October" Hospital; on January 1, 1942 only 27 physicians remained. Two died and two others became ill through exhaustion. Most of the remaining 23 were suffering from exhaustion as well, and the majority of them also had nutritional edema. Out of the medium-level personnel, 9 died of exhaustion in the course of 4 months.For reasons of hunger and disease 67 people were released from their duties, out of the personnel comprising 163 people. The large majority of the rest 96 people who were still functioning, were heavy dystrophics with edema. In the same 4 months, 23 members of the junior personnel died; by February 1, 1942, 93 had been released because of hunger. Seventy of 170 workers suffered from alimentary dystrophy. All stokers, attendants of the casualty ward, and grounds keepers of the hospital died of hunger during the same period [322]. Thus, the medical personnel themselves were badly in need of medical aid and nutrition.

These facts have not lost their relevance, even today. On the contrary, the experience leads us to reflect on what must be done and how, in a situation similar to that of Leningrad under siege, no matter whether the extreme conditions are brought on by war or by natural disaster. Without such foresight, such a situation cannot be handled effectively.

The lesson of Leningrad shows an absence of forethought. At the beginning of the war between the Soviet Union and Germany, nobody anticipated the possibility of blockade and famine. The ensuing course of military events, however, should have obliterated any initial optimism, and plans should have been made for a mass evacuation of women, children, the ill, and the aged. But insufficient information on the actual military situation and erroneous estimation of the prospects allowed for a passive attitude. Though it had been planned to evacuate 250 000 people between July 13 and 17, 1941 (i.e., 62 500 daily), only 49 400 were in fact sent away, i.e., 19.8% of the number planned. Moreover, the rate of evacuation was reduced because the municipal authorities had no vehicles available to transport the people to the various destinations [323]. At the same time, some trains left the city almost empty, carrying 8–10 people per coach [324].

The evacuation had not been properly planned from the beginning. During the period from June 29 to August 27, 1941, 395 091 children were evacuated. Of these, 175 400 were sent to the eastern and southeastern regions of the Leningrad district itself; upon approaching the site of military activities they were brought back into the city [325, p. 33].

Evacuation was continued during the blockade. Until January 22, 1942, people were leaving the city by crossing Lake Ladozhskoye, for the most part not in organized transport columns but on foot. Between the end of December 1941 and January 22, 1942, a total of 36 118 people were sent away from the city [325, p. 34]. In the period following – until April 15 – 480 000 people were transported by rail from Finland Station to Borisova Griva; 62 218 reached Borisova Griva by other means of transport and 11 968 on foot [325, p. 35].

Because of the hunger and the cold, casualties among the evacuated were high, as can be seen from Table 28, based on data from the Tikhvinsk evacuation point for the winter of 1942 [326]. Of the deaths, 62% were caused by alimentary dystrophy, 25.8% by infectious diseases, and 6.1% by pneumonia and heart disease. Thus, not only was the situation in Leningrad itself bad, but medical provision for the evacuees was also far from satisfactory. The reasons for this were:

1. Unjustifiable failure to create and maintain food reserves for emergency situations and to carry out a timely evacuation of the civilian population
2. Absence of a plan to provide food and emergency medical aid

Table 28. Some mortality data from Tikhvinsk evacuation center, winter 1942

Cause	n	%
Alimentary dystrophy	263	62
Intestinal infection	102	24
Wounds, trauma	25	6
Pneumonia	20	5
Heart disease	5	1
Dyspepsia	5	1
Epidemic typhus	2	<1
Infectious jaundice	2	<1
Others	2	<1
Total	426	

3. The sudden onslaught of widespread hunger under conditions of fall and winter cold
4. The extremely cruel military actions of the war, based as they were on the confrontation of two extreme ideologies
5. The upsetting of everyday life in a large modern city

With regard to point 5 above, I mean the malfunctioning of the water supply, the sewage system, central heating, energy supply, communication lines, transportation, and other modern services which have become routine. This does not mean merely inconveniences; in a situation of hunger and under unfavorable climatic conditions, this means high mortality in a short period of time.

Excluding the particular military and potentical factors, the data on besieged Leningrad can also serve to illustrate the public health consequences of widespread hunger as a natural disaster of a local character. We observe

a) a short transition period between the stages of malnutrition and hunger;
b) the grave effects of neuropsychological and physical stress and of the cold;
c) drastic increases in morbidity and mortality, with complications in diseases of the lungs (pneumonia, tuberculosis) and the gastrointestinal tract, and hypertensive and psychogenic illnesses; and
d) a drastic decrease in the birth rate and an unusual increase in mortality (initially for men, later for women), expressed as a negative population growth rate.

There is a certain degree of predetermination and regularity in situations such as those described. However, in the case of famine caused by a natural disaster, certain differences are observed, particularly with regard to its territorial extent. This is summarized in Table 29. The main differences are in the course and extent of the famine, the conditions under which help can be provided, and the particular public health consequences. These differences determine what measures should be taken to aid the stricken population.

It must be noted that, on the basis of available materials, provisions for combating famine and its consequences at present are unsatisfactory throughout the world. The essential difficulties are the biosocial factors, which are of a global nature. The direct result of this gloomy situation is that the first victims are children, and famine thus undermines the health and potential of the next generation. In India, malnutrition is widespread, affecting 13% of pregnant women and 21.9% of school children. It is estimated that by the year 2001 about 20% of India's population will be suffering from malnutrition [174]. In Iraq malnutrition is assumed to be the main cause of child mortality [181].

These facts must be considered in connection with the population explosion. The population of China in 1840 was 400 million. By the early 1950s it had exceeded 600 million. By 1969, a period of only 15 years, this figure was 800 million, and a further increase of 200 million was registered 11 years later [297].

Thus, the problems of malnutrition and hunger are interconnected with socioeconomic disorder in a country, lack of ecological balance, the tendency to generate and propagate cycles of destruction, and the population explosion. As a disaster having both natural and anthropogenic causes, hunger certainly poses problems to health security. These problems need to be solved on both the global and the national level, and the principal approach must be prevention.

Table 29. Comparative characteristics of local and widespread hunger

	Appearance	Territory	Aid	Evacuation	Refugees	Increase of morbidity			Increase of mortality	Natural movement of population
						General	Infectious	Psychical		
Wide-spread hunger	Slow, of long duration	Extensive	Determined by resources available	Possible	Masses	Mass	Mass, wide-spread	Considerable	Considerable	Considerable prevalence of deaths over births
Local hunger	Relatively rapid, of short duration	Limited	Limited or impossible	Impossible	Limited	Mass	Mass, local	Considerable	Considerable	Considerable prevalence of death over births

Public Health Consequences of Road Traffic Catastrophes

Road traffic catastrophes, which can involve many people and cause great sociohygienic and economic damage, are anthropogenic disasters. In many countries damage caused by traffic accidents exceeds that from earthquakes, floods, tsunami, and other calamities of natural origin.

The main causes of road disasters are closely connected with the problems relating to the ecological crisis, and to our modern way of life. Abbou [1], in considering the consequences of pollution and other harmful environmental effects, identifies the road catastrophe as one of the modern diseases determined by calamities of a mass nature.

Man seems to have lost control. Developments have become almost unmanageable. Technological progress has penetrated into all spheres of modern life. Mankind is dangerously close to becoming a captive of technology, the dictator [66, 244]. All this is occurring in a period of groping for new ethical, moral, and cultural values with which to lead civilization into the next century.

The process of urbanization increases the harm being done to the environment and the danger of road accidents. United Nations' documents indicate that the proportion of the world population that is urban increased from 26% in 1950 to 36% in 1970. In 1975 this index was 39% and it is envisaged that by the year 2000 half of the world's population will live in big cities [154]. At the same time, there is a discrepancy between the exploitation of the technical potential of roads and means of transportation on the one hand, and the requirements of speed, security of movement, parking facilities, and clean air on the other. In accommodating the demand for transportation there is frequently no consideration of:

1. Medicogeographical conditions (composition and character of the population, relief, extreme temperatures and atmospheric factors
2. Rational and efficient building and use of highways and roads, security of movement, and maximal provision for decongestion of main urban roads and intersections
3. The psychophysiological stress caused by the accelerated rhythm of life, and by personal and social relations which seem far from regulated

The essential obstacles to the solution of these morbid problems of modern city life are socioeconomic disorder and the ecological crisis. Small countries have an especially difficult time coping, as they bear heavy economic and energy burdens and face the migration of a considerable portion of their population.

The total number of automobiles in Israel increased 2.5 times in the course of 10 years (1965–1975), while the total number of kilometers covered by road vehicles increased 3 times. By 1985 the number of automobiles there will have reached 900 000, double that in 1975. There has been a corresponding increase in road traffic accidents. The situation is made worse by the fact that a large proportion of roads in Israel are urban (54%, as compared with 32% in England and 16% in the United States). Other small countries have similar problems. In Jamaica, mortality due to road traffic accidents increased from 421 victims per 100 000 vehicles in 1961 to 530 in 1970 [98].

To a certain extent, road traffic accidents have come to be viewed as an inevitable evil. They increase with the industrial and economic development of a country and the improvement of the standard of living. In the USA, road accidents killed 56 300 and injured 2 500 000 in 1972, and – as in Canada – were the leading cause of death for people aged between 1 and 37 years [86].

The public health consequences of road catastrophes account for a large portion of overall morbidity and mortality. In Israel (1975), traffic accidents were the seventh leading cause of death, after ischemic heart disease, cerebrovascular disease, various cancers, and accidents not connected with road vehicle travel. The projected annual mortality due to traffic accidents (for 1975) exceeded that for all other causes for men aged 1–70 and women aged 1–75 [209]. This picture is typical for other countries as well. On Taiwan within the period 1960–1977, accidents moved from seventh place among the causes of death to third. Most of these were road accidents, for 38.5% of women and 43.4% of men [228].

The fact that young people and children are involved in road accidents is of special concern. Not seldom, whole families are killed. In the United States, half of those between the ages of 1 and 14 years who die, do so from injuries, most of them incurred in road accidents [131].

Data from the World Health Organization and the European Economic Community reflecting the situation in 30 countries for the periods 1950–1954 and 1970–1974 show that in three-fourth of these countries the increased mortality due to road traffic accidents was disproportionately high for the group aged 15–24, for youth of both sexes, and for men [114].

It must also be noted that subjective factors exerted considerable influence on this mortality. In Israel, 80% of traffic accidents have behavioral origins; only 3%–4% are the result of organic diseases [265]. A special role is played by alcohol consumption. In Canada, 70% of male victims of traffic accidents aged 16–35 were intoxicated with alcohol [86]. In Jamaica, the corresponding figure was 45% [98].

The Chronicle of the World Health Organization (1969) states that persons with antisocial episodes in their life histories comprise a larger proportion of drivers who have been involved in traffic accidents than of those who have never been involved. They are more aggressive, and consequently more inclined to violate traffic regulations [116]. Thus, the drivers' behavior becomes the decisive causative factor of road accidents and of the injuries suffered in them. Since this information is available for registration and control, the role of the authorities responsible for health services becomes more important.

To a great extent, the psychic and the physical states of the driver predetermine the functioning of his decision-making capacity. This is especially critical in a situation which may bring the driver to a state of mental imbalance. Errors in apprehension of the situation and processing of the information are the main cause of 30%–60% of road accidents [210]. This makes it imperative to focus attention on psychophysiological testing, in order to determine a driver's capacity for apprehending a critical traffic situation and his ability to make the appropriate decisions.

Experience shows that psychic deviations are more dangerous to the driver than are somatic disturbances. Sudden attacks of various diseases account for only 1–2 accidents per 1000. In Sweden, for example, an experiment showed that the proportion of ill people among drivers involved in road accidents was only half as high as that in the control group [117]. The driver suffering from a somatic disease is likely to be more responsible for his actions and to have a highly developed self-discipline. He apprehends the risk of an accident which could not only complicate the course of his disease, but also bring about an irreversible catastrophe for those involved. It has been observed that drivers aged 65 and more are proportionately less involved in road accidents. This is the result of cautiousness, which goes hand in hand with experience and age, in apprehending the risks involved.

Health is a dynamic factor. A driver should be required to undergo

a) a comprehensive medical examination as part of the initial licensing procedure, and
b) systematic medical examinations at regular intervals.

Implementation of such measures is one aspect of the health services' activities aimed at preventing traffic accidents and the injuries they cause. However, the driver himself remains the one responsible for an accident.

Another important aspect is improvement of the general environmental situation. Activities to this end would be:

1. Research on the causes of road accidents and the character of the injuries they cause
2. Public health campaigns to combat bad habits such as consumption of alcohol and use of narcotics, as well as various antisocial inclinations such as aggressiveness
3. Urban planning; development of the road network in accordance with the needs of industry, the economy, culture, domestic services, population movement, and security in emergency situations

An important sociohygienic factor is the time of day the accident takes place. This has a bearing on the neuro-psycho-physiological capacities of the driver as far as

a) increase or decrease in the reactive state,
b) decrease in attention and in visual and auditory perception as a result of overtiredness or disturbed mental balance, and
c) his or her degree of individual discipline, moral and cultural behavior, and personal responsibility for other people and society at large.

Our modern way of life also plays an important role in accidents. For most people living in big cities it is common to be in a state of irritability and stress because of lack of recreation, constant haste on the way to and from work, bombardment by enormous amounts of information from radio, TV and the press, noise and air pollution, irregular mealtimes, and the generally negative effects of the sedentary life.

One's attention is captured by the absence of pedestrians in the streets of big cities in the United States and other countries, especially in the evenings. The endless flow of cars, resembling a conveyor belt, fills the streets, leaving behind polluted air. People sit in front of television sets or pursue other entertainment which requires no movement, instead of taking trips in the lap of nature, or walks in clear, green, and architecturally well-designed streets. All this exerts a bad influence on the behavior patterns of modern man, and, indirectly, upon traffic safety. Environmental sanitation is a direct concern of the public health authorities.

In the United States, more accidents occur between the hours of 10 and 12 a.m. than in any other 2-h period. Among the casualties who are children, infants (up to 1 year old) prevail (62% as compared with 29% of 1- to 14-year-olds). Older children are generally involved in the accidents which take place between 6 p.m. on Friday and midnight Sunday [131]. These figures are obviously predetermined by the style of life and activities of the American people. People in other countries show their own behavioral peculiarities. Extreme climatic and atmospheric conditions and mountainous countryside exert an influence on accidents as well.

Table 30 classifies traffic accidents in Israel according to the time of day they occur and the gravity of the injuries sustained [36]. Most accidents occur in the morning (6 to 11 a.m. – 30%) and in the afternoon (noon to 5 p.m. – 40%). There is a marked decrease in the evening (6 to 11 p.m. – 23%) and especially at night (midnight to 5 a.m. – 6%–7%), though the gravity of nighttime accidents increases; the rates of killed and injured are 9% and 8.2% respectively. At night drivers are less attentive and less observant of traffic regulations, and are more inclined to exceed the speed limit. So the subjective factors are decisive – tiredness, loss of reactive capacity, attitudes toward road and vehicle conditions.

As roads within municipal boundaries comprise the major portion of the Israeli traffic network, there is an increase in accidents involving pedestrians, especially at crossroads, coincident with increased traffic intensity

a) at midday (11 to 1),
b) at the time when children are returning from school, and
c) during the afternoon rush hour (3–5 p.m.).

Traffic accidents occurring at these times comprise 6.9% of the total and account for 7.1% of the killed and 7.2% of the seriously injured.

On public holidays in every country, including the day before and the day after, traffic is especially dense and especially dangerous. The subjective factors, rooted in the local peculiarities of the specific population, predominate among the causes. This is illustrated in Fig. 26, which provides a weekly specification of those injured in road accidents in Israel [36]. The highest proportion of injuries (16.2%) are incurred on the first day of the week (Sunday); this is also the case for deaths resulting from traffic accidents (16%). From here on, up to Thursday, the fifth day of the week, the proportions tend to decrease. The weekend (Friday and Saturday) shows a continuance of this tendency in absolute figures (14.1% and 11.6% injured), while the percentage killed then is 12.4% and 11.9%. But since the intensity of traffic on these 2 days is the lowest for the week in Israel (excluding the Friday afternoon and Sunday evening hours), the percentage of injuries and the consequent mortality must be considered relatively high. Subjective factors here may be the possible

Table 30. Road traffic casualties by gravity of injuries and time when incurred, Israel, 1978 (%)

Casualties \ Hour of day	Morning						Afternoon						Evening						Night						Unknown
	06	07	08	09	10	11	12	13	14	15	16	17	18	19	20	21	22	23	24	01	02	03	04	05	
Total	4.1	5.6	5.0	4.6	4.9	5.7	6.5	6.9	6.8	6.4	6.7	6.9	5.7	4.9	4.2	3.2	2.4	2.6	1.6	1.2	0.8	0.5	0.6	1.6	
	29.9						40.2						23.0						6.3						0.6
Killed	4.7	3.7	4.0	5.7	3.7	4.7	5.7	7.8	6.3	6.6	5.0	7.1	5.8	6.6	3.4	3.7	1.9	2.6	0.9	0.9	0.6	1.1	1.1	4.4	
	26.5						38.5						24.0						9.0						2.0
Severely injured	4.2	4.7	4.1	4.3	4.7	5.0	5.9	6.8	6.3	6.8	6.7	7.2	6.0	5.2	4.7	3.2	3.2	2.2	2.2	1.8	0.9	0.7	0.7	1.9	
	27.0						39.7						24.5						8.2						0.6
Slightly injured	3.6	5.8	5.6	4.6	5.1	5.9	6.7	6.9	6.9	6.3	6.8	6.8	5.6	4.8	4.1	3.2	2.3	2.7	1.5	1.1	0.7	0.5	0.6	1.4	
	30.6						40.4						22.7						5.8						0.5

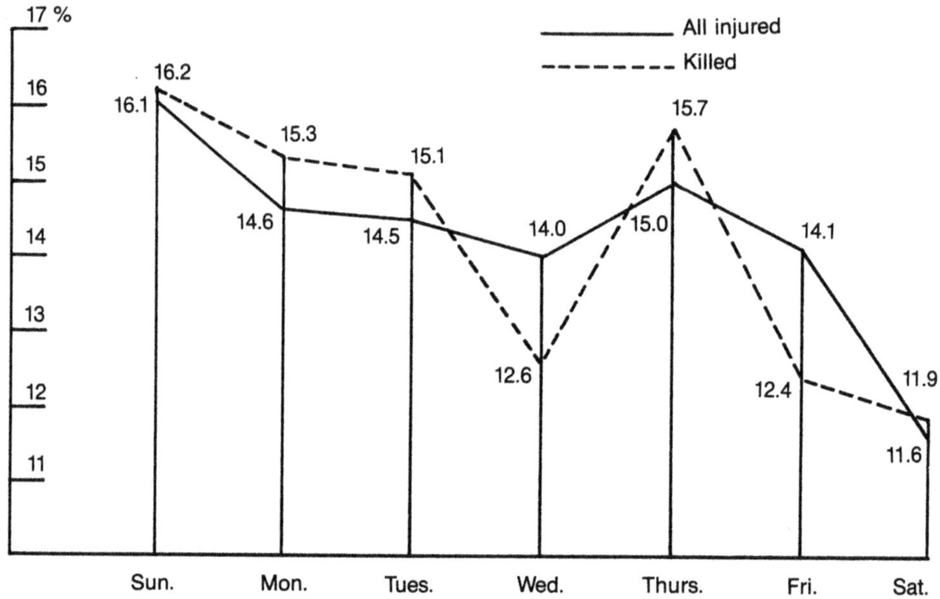

Fig. 26. Breakdown of road traffic casualties by days of the week, Israel 1978 [36]

impact of alcohol, narcotics, or medication, and the peculiarities of character and habits of recreation. To these must be added the stimulation of war and individual misfortunes.

These factors can produce errors in perception and processing of traffic information. Among the objective factors are drastic changes in temperature and atmospheric conditions. Fig. 27 [36] indicates an increase of injuries due to traffic accidents in July and August in Israel (8.9%–9.6%) and a resulting high mortality (10.5%–11.5%). This period of the year corresponds to the season of leaves and festive days in Israel, which is naturally connected with increased traffic. But there is another reason for an increase in accidents at this time: this is the season with the highest temperatures and with intensive sun, and these influence the reactive state and behavior of drivers. What is meant here is the observed syndrome of hysteria in men and the asthenic-hyperdynamic syndrome in women in hot countries [22].

Another increase in accidents and injuries in Israel is indicated for October–November, when drastic changes in temperature and atmospheric conditions in mountainous areas bring about changes in driving conditions on the one hand, and errors by both drivers and pedestrians on the other – both with grave consequences.

Certain roads marked by dense traffic and specific conditions are especially dangerous. In Israel, 65% of all traffic incidents occur on only 15% of the country's roads [36]. These roads are in areas of dense population and high concentration of industrial, financial, cultural, and entertainment institutions and are distinguished by a faster, more intense pace of life. The largest city, Tel Aviv, is situated at the center of the country's highway network and constitutes a gigantic national crossroads.

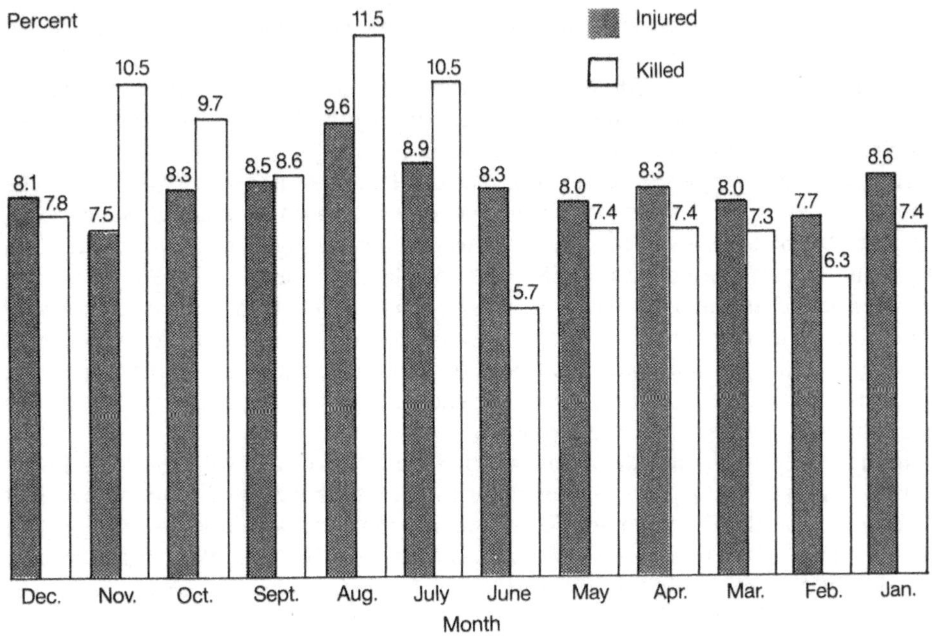

Fig. 27. Breakdown of road traffic casualties by months of the year, Israel 1978 [36]

Involvement in road accidents is different for men and women, for drivers and pedestrians, and for people of different ages; measures undertaken to reduce the number of accidents must take these differences into consideration. Statistics from the Haifa area show that drivers comprised 37.8%, passengers 31.5%, and pedestrians 30.7% of those involved in traffic accidents [36]. In Japan, 57% of those killed or injured in accidents were drivers and 23% pedestrians. In addition, under the specific conditions in Tokyo, pedestrians comprised 45% of the total killed, 32.3% of them on the *sidewalks* [133]. The reasons are evidently the extreme density of the traffic, especially at crossroads, and the failure to observe traffic regulations.

Men prevail among the injured; in the Haifa area the proportions were 67.6% men, 32.4% women [36]. Corresponding data from Canada show that men are injured in traffic accidents 1.5 times as often as women [110]. In Austria in 1979 there were 2.24 thousand deaths from traffic accidents; of these, 1.69 thousand were men and 0.55 thousand were women [274], i.e., three times as many men as women. To a great extent, of course, this proportional difference is due to the fact that the majority of drivers are men. In addition, women drivers are less involved in alcohol consumption, use of narcotics, and other antisocial activities; they tend to be more cautious and more responsible drivers.

There are more private vehicles than public vehicles involved in traffic accidents. In Israel, 59.1% of vehicles involved in accidents are private cars and only 11.9% buses and taxis [36]. Therefore, a well-planned development of public transportation which considers the needs of the population in question is the best way to reduce the number of accidents and injuries. Such development must, of course, go hand in hand with environmental sanitation. The social significance of such measures increases daily. According to the growth dynamics of traffic accidents (relevant for 1977), the situation is most dangerous in South Africa. Following this are Greece, Norway, and the Federal Republic of Germany.

In Israel, 9545 people were killed in the four Israeli-Arab wars (1948–1973). The number killed in road accidents during the 10-year period of 1968–1978 was 6553, i.e., 68.6% of the figure for the four wars. The number of people injured in accidents in this period was 37 389, and of slightly injured, 183 590. The ratio between killed and injured was 1:34. In fact, road traumatism in Israel is not very much less than war traumatism, and may be considered a traumatic epidemic of peacetime. Aid for such large numbers of injured becomes a complex problem, involving preventive measures, medical and emergency aid at the scene of the accident, and evacuation of the injured.

In order to provide aid, the nature of the injuries associated with traffic accidents must be known. To this end, S. Beinin elaborated materials from 400 road accident cases treated at the Rambam and Rotschield hospitals of Haifa in 1979–1980 [36]. Of the patients, 281 were men (70.3%) and 119 women (29.7%). With regard to age, the distribution was as follows: 0–4 years, 21 (5.3%); 5–14 years, 68 (17%); 15–64 years, 282 (70.5%); 65 years and older, 29 (7.2%). The general structure of the injuries is shown in Table 31 [36]; the bulk of the victims (65.6%) had head injuries. In 30.8% of these cases the head injuries were combined with others. Skull traumas can be classified as medium or severe. The severe cases involved fractures of the fornix or base of the skull, internal cranial hemorrhage, heavy contusions, and commotio cerebri. They were always accompanied by loss of or disturbances in consciousness. Head contusions were registered in 3% of cases.

Cases of commotio cerebri alone accounted for 30% of the total cases of head injuries accompanied by commotio cerebri, while those accompanied by skull fractures comprised 28% of the total number of head injuries. The latter contingent of patients constituted extremely difficult cases, because of the need for a life-saving regime during evacuation from the site of the accident.

Commotio cerebri combined with multiple fractures of the body and the extremities comprised 23% of the total number of head injuries. In addition to life-

Table 31. Single and multiple locations of injuries as proportions of total hospitalized as a result of road traffic accidents, Haifa (1979–1980)

	Single location (n)	Proportion (%)	Multiple location (n)	Proportion (%)	Combined (n)	Proportion (%)
Head	139	34.8	123	30.8	262	65.5
Thorax	8	2.0	69	17.3	77	19.3
Abdominal organs	3	0.8	20	5.0	23	5.8
Spine	5	1.3	15	3.8	20	5.0
Pelvis and pelvic organs	5	1.3	35	8.8	40	10.0
Extremities	40	10.0	88	22.0	128	32.0
Soft tissues	21	5.3	89	22.3	110	27.5

Single location, n = 221 (55.3%); Multiple location, n = 179 (44.7%); Total, n = 400

saving first aid, these patients required immobilization of the extremities in order to prevent a state of deep shock, or to make the course of shock easier. In 4% of head injury cases, commotio cerebri was combined with damages to vital internal organs. These included the cardiovascular system and the lungs (hemorrhages). In such cases, reanimation at the site of the accident is of prime importance. Five percent of head injuries involve injuries to the eyes [36]. Such patients require evacuation to special hospitals.

Injuries to the head are the most common type in road accidents. The head is the least protected part of the body. The danger of contusion and commotio cerebri is increased by the fact that loss of consciousness causes the driver to lose steering control.

The actual timing of the effects of an injury can vary, for they can be both immediate and delayed. They can also be temporary or permanent. This determines the degree of disablement. It is clear, then, that the development of optimally protective headgear for drivers is important. Such a helmet should meet the requirements for efficient protection, lightness, and convenience.

Next in scope to head injuries are injuries to the extremities; 22% of these are combined with other injuries. Cases accompanied by damage to main vessels are most dangerous. This complicates the system of medical aid and evacuation, as the primary function of first aid is to help at the site of the accident and to prevent shock.

The type of first aid administered depends on the localization and combination of injuries. Fig. 28 [36] illustrates the large portion of fractures of the lower extremities (61%), excluding those of upper and lower limbs combined. Closed fractures comprise 84% of extremities fractures, and combined fractures of upper and lower extremities occur in 12% of cases, and comprise 32% of the total number of cases hospitalized.

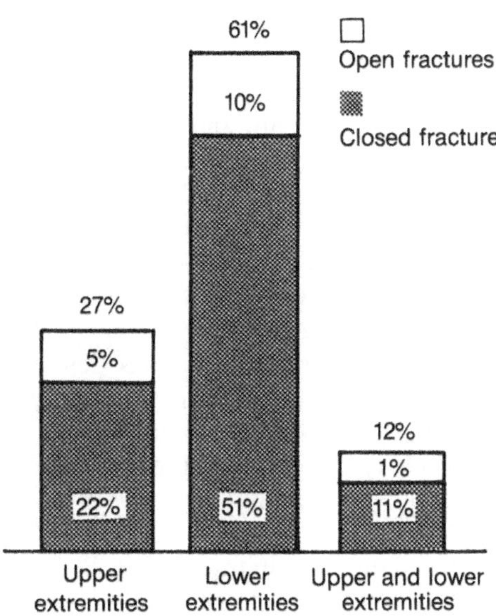

Fig. 28. Breakdown of extremities fractures incurred in road traffic catastrophes, Israel [36]

Open fractures comprise 16% of fractures of the extremities. Patients with such fractures need transport immobilization and administration of analgesics at the site of the accident. Unfortunately, through poor planning, these measures are often not available.

Third in place, after injuries to the head and the extremities are those to the soft tissues (27.5%), 22.3% of which are combined with other injuries. Extensive injuries to soft tissues cause painful irritation and toxemia, i.e., absorption of toxic products from the crushed tissues, and thus are distinguished by their extremely severe course.

Of the total number of injuries in road accidents, 19.3% are to the thorax; 17.3% of patients hospitalized had combined thorax injuries. According to Soviet authors [260], 49.7% of trauma cases connected with the thorax are accompanied by injuries to one other part of the body; 37% with injuries to two other parts of the body; 11% with three; 5.7% with four; 1.2% with five; and 0.5–0.7% with injuries to six or seven other parts of the body.

Combined traumas to the head and thorax are the most severe. Penetrating injuries to the thorax have a high mortality. More than any others, this contingent of patients needs urgent, specialized aid at the site of the accident. Combined traumas to the thorax and the abdomen comprise 23% of cases [260]. Traumas to organs of the thorax (61.6%) occur in these patients much more than in isolated pure thoracic traumas (28.2%). The most frequent cases are rib fractures.

In cases of thoracic injuries, the gravity of the situation, the extent and nature of medical aid provided, and the order and means of evacuation all depend on whether the injuries are accompanied by

a) damage to internal organs and bones;
b) closed/open pneumothorax;
c) disturbances in the functioning of vital organs;
d) shock and loss of blood.

In thoracoabdominal injuries, internal loss of blood is the main cause of death.

From the viewpoint of the gravity of their consequences, injuries to the head, and to the head and thorax combined account for a large proportion of road accident casualties (both death and disability). Safety improvements in vehicles and protective gear for the head, thorax, and other vital parts of the body are needed.

Injuries to the pelvis and its organs require specific medical aid at the site of the accident. They make up 10% of the injuries in traffic accidents, and are mostly closed in nature. In 8.8% of cases these injuries are combined with others. Pelvic injuries include wounds and closed pelvic fractures, frequently accompanied by shock. According to Soviet authors [260], 16% of pelvic injuries are combined with those of the thorax. All victims delivered to hospitals show traumatic shock, and mortality is 31%. This is explained by insufficient medical aid at the site of the accident and delayed evacuation.

Injuries to the abdominal cavity comprise 5.8% [36]. In penetrating injuries, the organs most commonly damaged are the liver and the spleen. The retroperitoneal organs are damaged in 3% of cases. In 75% of cases with nonpenetrating abdominal injuries there are injuries as well to the head, thorax and/or extremities [36]. Multiple injuries to the skull, thorax, pelvis and pelvic organs, and to the bones and joints of the extremities comprise 15% of cases. The grave condition of those with penetrating abdominal wounds is caused by shock and internal hemorrhaging. To a great extent their lives depend on how fast emergency medical aid is provided at the accident site.

Most characteristic of the injuries caused by traffic accidents are internal abdominal traumas with damage (ruptures) to the internal organs: liver, spleen, kidneys, intestines. The clinical picture of these cases resembles that of abdominal injuries incurred in war [258].

This detailed discussion of specific injuries caused by traffic accidents is aimed at the following:

1. Improved construction of vehicles to increase driver and passenger security, and the search for means of protection of the individual against traumas in road accidents
2. Special drivers' training in the elements of first aid for traumatic injuries and reanimation, including: bandaging of wounds and burns, temporary stopping of bleeding; immobilization of fractured extremities and severely damaged soft tissue; closed-chest massage and artificial ventilation of the lungs by the mouth-to-mouth and mouth-to-nose methods; and correct and efficient removal of the injured from destroyed, burning, or overturned vehicles, if no trained rescue team is present
3. Preparedness to provide emergency and specialized medical aid at the site of an accident at any moment

Points 1 and 2 above deal with prevention on the part of the public health authorities and drivers themselves; the passing of an examination on medical assistance should be included in the requirements for receiving a driver's license, as should a comprehensive examination of the driver's health. Such training of drivers would increase the efficiency of medical aid provided at the site of accidents. It might also exert a favorable influence on the behavior of the individual driver and reduce the number of road accidents that are due to subjective factors.

In terms of sanitation of the environment, road traffic accidents are only part of a much larger problem. A practical solution of this is within the reach of any country. It depends on:

1. Development of a communication network with alternatives, taking into consideration the local geographical, hydrological, climatic, and meteorological factors in their extreme manifestations
2. The character and way of life of the population; the relative involvement of drivers and pedestrians in road accidents
3. Prevention of air pollution, and planning and development of urban areas and highways with a view to prevention of accidents and fast evacuation
4. Planning for emergency rescue in the case of natural disasters
5. Public health education concerning natural disasters in general and traffic accidents in particular, with the cooperation of police and the media

Factors Predetermining the Method of Eliminating the Public Health Consequences of Natural Disasters

With respect to the organization of a system of medical aid provision and to the methods of remedying public health consequences, the various forms of natural disasters involve the same considerations. These include:

1. Area of distribution, time of appearance, and gravity and duration of the injurious effects
2. The situation in the stricken area, with regard to the phases and their duration, the manifestation of stress, and the general structure and nature of the injuries
3. The impact of particular geographical conditions
4. The preparedness of the public health authorities for emergency situations
5. The reasons for injurious effects and their universal character, and their impact on the country's social and political health

Natural disasters appear suddenly. Affecting large areas, they have great impact on populations and environments. The everyday way of life of the area, shaped slowly over many years, suddenly changes. The combined effect of several natural disasters, differing in origin and character (earthquakes, tsunami, floods, mudflows, avalanches), sometimes takes on the proportions of a cataclysm. Changes occur in topographical relief, soil, river flows. The Chilean people, for instance, encountered such a catastrophe in May 1960, and catastrophic quakes lasted in Turkey from December 26, 1939 till January 2, 1940. One-sixth of the territory of Turkey suffered because of them. On December 31, 1939 there was also a strong tsunami in the western part of the country, and floods enveloped the Black Sea coast [108]. The scope of the injuries and the gravity of the situation made it impossible for the authorities in Chile and Turkey to cope without external help.

Even relatively small disasters can have grave consequences. On May 14, 1970 an earthquake registered 8 on the Richter scale struck one-quarter of Daghestan (USSR), affecting 50% of the republic's population. It caused avalanches and landslides in the mountains. Twenty-two settlements were destroyed and 257 others were partially damaged. Most severely hit were the towns of Bujnaksk, Makhachkala, and Kiziljurt. Hospitals, schools, children's institutions, and office buildings housing public services were put out of action. Prolonged torrents brought floods lasting for 2 weeks [56, 252]. The fact that the disasters followed each other in rapid succession aggravated the situation. The combined effects brought about a crisis in the places with the least resistance (locus minoris resistentia). They also hindered emergency rescue operations, medical aid to the injured, and a quick return to acceptable public health conditions.

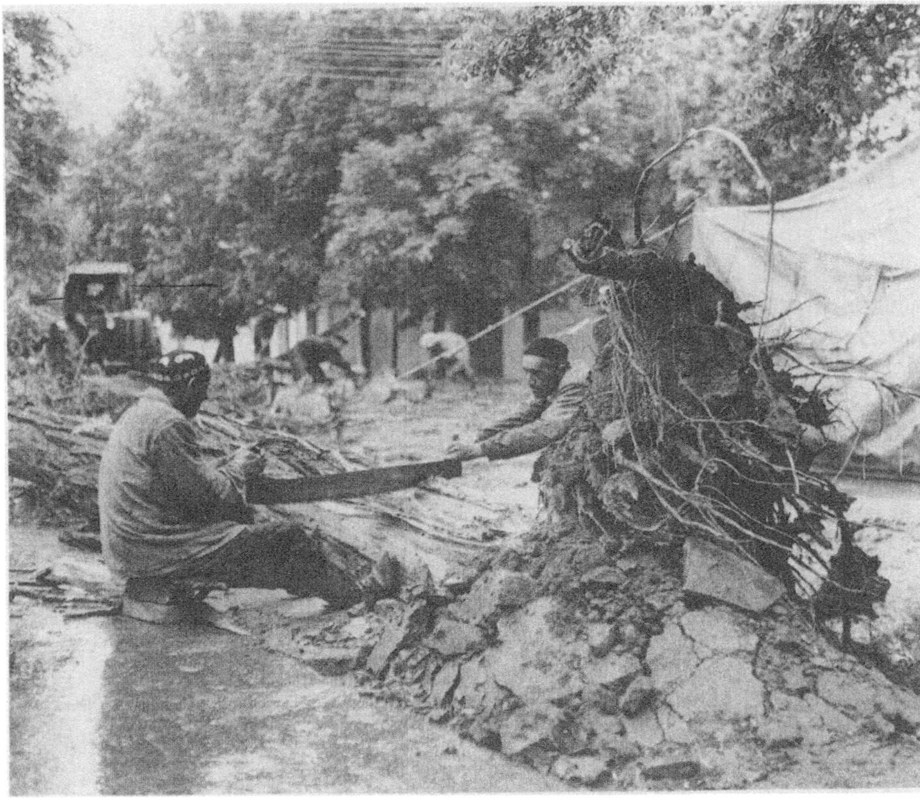

Fig. 29. Trees uprooted by hurricane, Tashkent, May 5, 1966 (Photo R. Shemutdinov)

The duration of a natural disaster defies prediction. The epicenter of the magnitude-8 earthquake in Tashkent (April 16, 1966) devastated an area of 10 km^2. For an entire year thereafter, 800 underground tremors appeared periodically in full swing, 38 of them reaching magnitude 5. Recurring magnitude-7 tremors took place on May 10 and 24 and June 5 and 29, 1966, and again on March 25, 1967 [157]; they were of relatively short duration. This caused and maintained high tension, bringing about a succession of injuries. As if to test the situation, a hurricane struck Tashkent on May 5, 1966, uprooting trees (Fig. 29) and tearing down tents in which the injured were being treated after having been evacuated from the destroyed hospitals and in which those left homeless had found shelter.

This picture is not unique. It describes the unstable situation at the site of any natural disaster. There are many – often unpredictable – factors involved. The latent power of nature comes to the fore insidiously, gradually accumulating to a critical point, at which it manifests as an extreme phenomenon with devastating effects.

If no efficient system of protection has been organized, the result is all the worse. Preparation for possible disaster, supervision and control of protective materials (used for various purposes in everyday life), can do much to reduce the gravity of the consequences.

There are three periods distinguishable with regard to a natural disaster:

1. The beginning, lasting for approximately 24 h
2. The period in which damages and injuries become manifest (including secondary injuries caused by fires, crashes, floods, etc.), lasting from several days up to a month or more
3. The elimination of the consequences, including those to public health, lasting up to a year or more

Each of these periods has its characteristic problems and conditions for their solution, which in turn determine the duration of the disaster. The medicosanitary characteristics of the damaged area according to these periods are presented in Table 32. Special attention should be paid to the stress reaction. In the first period especially, there is considerable stress on those involved in providing aid, particularly medical aid. Fright and horror can lead to panic. Deussen [58, 59, 60] states that

Table 32. Public health of natural disasters

	Immediate period	Intermediate period	Longer term
Events	Catastrophe	Secondary catastrophe	Return to equilibrium
Duration	1–24 h	approx. 1–30 days	30 days to > 1 year
Reaction to stress	Mass hysteria, panic	Depression	Neuroses
Injuries			
Traumas	Mass	Mass	Inconsiderable
Drownings (tsunami, floods, mudflows)	Mass	Sporadic	Irregular
Various (also due to secondary catastrophes)	Mass	Mass	Irregular
Diseases			
Somatic	Inconsiderable	Increasing	Still increasing
Infectious	Inconsiderable	Epidemic proportions esp. intestinal infections and children with infections	Sometimes still of epidemic proportions
Evacuation of			
Injured and diseased	Search, extraction, delivery to medical and evacuation points	Mass	Does not apply
Homeless	Guiding to centers for placement and evacuation	Mass	Does not apply
Geographic peculiarities	Impact of extreme temperature change	Rugged relief, destroyed communication lines make situation worse	Planned placement of new settlements, with regard to terrain and communication possibilities
Public health care/civil defense response	Emergency medical aid dispatched to victims	Implementation of treatment and prophylactic measures	Restoration of network of health services; elimination of longer term effects

panic is a common reaction for many people, whose disordered actions, though senseless, possess a great power of influence upon individuals who are not yet enveloped in the panic (the phenomenon of so-called psychic infection). Another attribute of panic is its neuropsychopathic character. According to Deussen, 11% of people show deviations from the psychic norm at least once in their lifetime. Especially endangered are people who suffer from mental illnesses such as schizophrenia; observation and control of these people and their timely evacuation are of utmost importance.

The primary psychological shock may last for half an hour. Later on, the stress reaction, which according to Hans Selye [229] functions as a protective mechanism, causes people to flee from the oncoming danger. After the Messina earthquake and tsunami (1908), crowds of almost naked residents rushed about the streets screaming for help. Fright paralyzes the will, badly affecting people's reason and behavior. Only 10%–20% of those in a disaster area act normally and with full senses; 10%–15% show complete helplessness [96]. After the 1940 earthquake in Tiraspol (USSR) I observed the inadequate activities of people trying to escape the danger. This resulted in injuries, in two cases ending in death. The situation after the Tashkent earthquake in 1966 was similar. It must be noted that the reactions and subsequent actions described here are characteristic of people living in areas which have more than once been hit by natural disasters.

When the earthquake (magnitude 6–7) of November 15, 1968 hit Ashkhabad, panic seized the people. The residents of Shorkala ran out of their houses, some jumping out of windows. The majority did not return to their homes for a long time. Some of those who jumped from second-floor windows were injured, and others fell in rushing down stairs. Panic spread to the neighboring settlements of Geok-Tepe, Colony, Yangikaly, and the health resort of Firjuza [99]. The roar of crashing buildings, the dust, the fires, the cries of desperate people, the weeping of children and women, the feeling of helplessness and doom – all of these add to the sense of horror. As Pablo Neruda has put it, there comes a "cosmic fright," the sudden loss of everything.

Nightfall aggravates the situation. Time seems endless. Then, when daylight comes showing the destruction, the suffering people, the killed and injured, and bringing with it the awareness of the loss of relatives and worldy goods, there is frequently a deep depression. This effect is characteristic of the third period of a disaster.

The stress reaction is also aggravated by traumatic injuries, environmental conditions, extremes of cold or heat, dust and mud, the absence of water, mass evacuations, and – in the case of earthquakes – repeated underground tremors. Such a situation renders people incapable of protecting themselves or assisting others. The local system of planned emergency rescue may be rendered ineffective because of damage, a discrepancy between the demands and the objective capabilities, and underestimation of natural and social factors which emerge under the disaster conditions (social conflict, criminality, anarchic behavior). For a certain period of time the possibility of loss of control cannot be ruled out; only extreme measures undertaken by external forces can change this situation.

Prolonged seismic activity can maintain long-term tension among people, without causing any injuries. The residents of Matsusiro (town, pop. 22 600, northwest of

Tokyo) experienced 300 000 separate tremors during one single year (1966). School children had to have their lessons in specially reinforced bunkers or tents. Many people slept fully clothed, ready for evacuation in case an earthquake occurred during the night [327].

When tsunami strike, many people are carried out into the ocean on planks, roofs, or other objects. The loneliness of these people aggravates their stress, even if it is not long before they are rescued. Lack of faith in the possibility of receiving external help adds to their problem. Many people are overcome by loneliness in any unfavorable situation. The fight for individual survival becomes extremely hard, affected as it is by

a) the victim's physical state;
b) climatic and meteorological conditions;
c) the duration of exposure in the open sea;
d) the need for means of flotation, food, and drinking water;
e) the possible need for medical care [31].

In speaking of people who are shipwrecked, Bombard [43] concludes that many die much earlier than the conditions really would indicate. Despair kills them before their physical forces are exhausted. This evidently also applies to those washed out to sea by tsunami.

During the third period, that of eliminating the public health consequences of the disaster, the stress reaction is also manifested as increased neuropsychological reactivity. Complications are observed in the course of disease, particularly in cardiovascular cases.

The geographical conditions of an area also influence the provision of medical aid and the return to order. Particular factors are

a) the unfavorable effects of both heat and cold;
b) the location of settlements and the communication between them;
c) mountainous relief and bodies of water.

Based on my personal experience, let us consider as a model of the above the extreme zones of Kamchatka and Central Asia (USSR). Though they differ greatly with regard to nature and climate, they resemble one another as regards the relatively frequent occurrence of various natural disasters.

The Kamchatka district, including the Komandor Islands, comprises 15% of the total land area of the USSR Far East territory, while its population constitutes only 5% of the total. It has a short, cold, and rainy summer, almost constant wind force 5–12 points in spring and autumn with extremely unstable weather and sharp diurnal temperature differences, and a long winter (October to late May). The temperature on the coldest days reaches –30°C. Snowdrifts are high, and the snow cover reaches 1 m and more. Prolonged (up to 7 days) and frequent snowstorms limit visibility and bring all road and air transportation to a standstill. The sea, however, never freezes over. Strong storms take place 4–6 times a month, from November to February, with wind force 5–10 points, frequently causing damage to coastal settlements.

Distribution of the population is connected with the internal water resources of the area and the surrounding seas. The majority of settlements are situated along rivers and on the coast. The distances between them are great, and communication is unsatisfactory. Along with relatively large settlements with populations exceeding 1000 there are many small ones. The population density of the vast Kamchatka territory, which exceeds that of many countries, is small (0.5–1.1/km^2). There is extensive migration among the people.

These geographical and demographic conditions pose difficulties in the allocation of public health services and in the provision of adequate medical care. In large settlements the network of medical, public health, and epidemiological institutions is relatively satisfactory, but people in smaller settlements are partly deprived of such services.

Personal observations and data provided by a typical district of Kamchatka (Ust-Bolsheretzky) for 1957 [32] lead to the conclusion that diseases of the respiratory tract constitute 50% of the general morbidity here; skin diseases follow at 18% and ear, nose, and throat problems at 10%. The main cause for this is the cooling factor combined with high humidity. Avtsyn [22] cites the significance of chronic, non-specific lung diseases in the northern regions, where low temperatures in both winter and summer combine with an extremely high humidity index. Especially negative is the role of strong winds; even reasonable external conditions become unbearable with high-speed winds, and they acquire a special significance during natural disasters.

Cardiovascular conditions among residents of the north take on a peculiar course. Avtsyn [22] distinguishes a special northern variation of hypertensive disease. The connection between wind with high humidity and morbidity due to heart disease has been revealed as being statistically reliable.

Thus, under northerly conditions, planning for medical aid and public health during natural disasters must take into consideration:

1. The cold climate combined with a high humidity index and frequent winds, regardless of season
2. The special character of pathology in the north, especially with regard to diseases of the respiratory tract and skin and cardiovascular disease
3. Peculiarities of mountain relief and bodies of water, which determine location of settlements, communication conditions, and manner of providing medical aid
4. Possible difficulties in getting rescue teams to the disaster site and in evacuating the injured; initial reliance on limited local forces and means

The extreme zone of Central Asia (USSR) is distinguished by its harsh climate. In the foothill areas and adjacent plains the summer is long, with temperatures exceeding +30°C; in certain places (such as the town of Termez) it reaches +50°C in the shade. Under such conditions a natural disaster can cause heat stress, which is especially dangerous for children.

The local dry winds (*garmsil* and *afganetz)* maintain extremely hot weather. Rising clouds of loess dust intensify the effect of the heat, making it unbearable. Strong winds blowing from the north, northwest, and west cause a sharp decrease in temperature and the summer nights are comparatively cool. The difference between the highest day and the lowest night temperature reaches an average of 15°–20°C.

The winter is relatively cold. The northeast winds bring strong frosts which last for 2–3 weeks.Spring is known for frequent torrential rains. Together with fast-melting snow and mountain glaciers they cause catastrophic floods on the Amu-Darja, Syr-Darja, and other rivers.

Mountains occupy a considerable part of Central Asia (in Tajikistan they comprise 90% of the total territory). The highest USSR mountain chains are found here (Pamirs and Badakhshan). Many Pamirs summits exceed 6000 m. Between the Ilijsk and Tajik valleys rises the huge Tien Shan mountain chain. Earthquakes connected with tectonic movements are relatively frequent in the mountains of Central Asia. Some territories (Pamirs, Badakhshan) are said to be vulnerable to quakes of magnitude 9–10.

Climatic conditions change with altitude. The summer is short, cool, and humid in the mountains; the severe winter lasts for 9 months. On the Tien Shan the temperature reaches only +5°– +6° C in June, and in the Pamirs, +14° C. During the day it undergoes drastic changes; e.g., a change from +33°C at 1 p.m. to –6.4° C at 4 p.m. was registered in the Pamirs [180]. Drastic changes in climatic conditions bring about considerable shifts of the thermoregulation process.

Much of the precipitation on the Tien Shan, Pamirs, and Badakhshan ranges comes in late spring and early summer. Not seldom, torrential rains cause mudflows, generally encountered in the Fergan valley.

The Central Asian settlements are situated mainly on the slopes and foothills, and in the river valleys. Though the avarage population density is $11/km^2$, it reaches $200–300/km^2$ in some valleys and in the intermountain plains. Most people live in easily destroyed clay buildings.

The specific geographical conditions of the Central Asian high-altitude regions (low temperatures, drastic changes in atmospheric pressure, high humidity, too little oxygen) add to the problems of a natural disaster. Destruction of mountain roads and highways limits access for emergency rescue teams, medical forces, and other types of aid to the stricken population and hampers evacuation. In the Gerushinsky and Sisiansky regions of Armenia, which were struck by an earthquake on May 2, 1931, 341 people died, 1000 were injured, and many thousands were made homeless [328]. The routes to the damaged settlements were blocked by rocks which had rolled down from the mountains; this delayed timely provision of aid to the injured, ill, and homeless. The situation in the Ordubatsky region was similar. By May 4, 1935, 67 killed and 573 injured were reported here; 13 000 people remainded in the open, exposed to rain and snow. All roads in the mountainous parts, and some of those in the plains had been destroyed [329].

The specific geographical conditions of Central Asia predetermine the local pathology. A considerable number of natural reservoirs of disease in the USSR have been registered in mountainous regions [48]. Avtsyn [21] assumes that the extreme zones of the mountains have the most unfavorable climatic effects on the human organism. Chief among the extremes is the heat. Regarding the pathology of the hot, arid zones of the USSR, Avtsyn [22] notes heat stroke and other manifestations of overheating, gastrointestinal diseases (especially among small children), and a wide distribution of certain parasitic infections. Hot climates are far more favorable for the spread of microbes than are moderate climates. The high rate of intestinal illness (infectious and noninfectious) in Central Asia is connected, according to Atakhanov [19], with the hot climate and its influence on the enzyme-secreting functions of the gastrointestinal tract, and with the high-carbohydrate diet.

Intestinal infections are not only more frequent here, but also more complicated. In the hot climate of Samarkand the course of typhoid is longer and more complicated than in more moderate areas. Complications and death are twice as frequent here than elsewhere. The hot climate inhibits the development and proper functioning of the patient's humoral and cellular immunity, causing complications, longer duration, and more frequent bacteriosis [4].

Of the group of typhoid-parathypoid patients tested in Tashkent, 4.4% were discovered to be carriers; 3.6% of typhoid patients and 7% of paratyphoid patients were carriers. Of the typhoid carriers, 5.6% were women and only 1.8% were men [141].

Given the favorable conditions for the spread of intestinal infections in Central Asia, and the greater vulnerability of women in earthquakes, the public health consequences of a natural disaster are grave indeed. Thus, in areas with geographical conditions similar to those in Central Asia, planning for the emergency situation which follows a natural disaster must consider the following factors:

1. Hot summer weather, effects of thermal stress, and those of wide ranges of diurnal temperature
2. The specific mountain relief, bodies of water, and desert conditions which determine the location of settlements, and the uneven population density
3. Hindrances to emergency rescue activities, provision of medical aid, and evacuation
4. Conditions favorable to the spread of intestinal diseases and those which multiply in polluted water

The severity of the situation in a stricken area obliges the authorities responsible for health services to assign the maximal available maneuverable forces and means to the area within the minimal amount of time. Public health services must be constantly prepared for such an emergency. The extent of such preparedness depends on:

1. How efficiently basic needs can be provided for
2. The public health-epidemiological situation in the period directly preceding the disaster
3. The organization, personnel, and equipment of the health services
4. The general cultural background of the population

The establishment of such an efficient system, and its capacity to meet the country's needs, depend on economic, historical, social, and political factors which are not the subject of this work. Point 2 above is of the utmost importance in an emergency situation. In the Ust-Bolsheretzky district on the west coast of Kamchatka, dysentery was a cause for concern in 1957. After the November 1957 flood, the incidence of dysentery increased by 44%, as reported by the Oktiabrsky district hospital [32]. The main reason for the increase was clearly the preceding unstable epidemiological state and the pollution of the territory's water supply due to the flood. This situation is not unique in the USSR.

According to reports from the Novgorod region public health institutions, the town of Chudovo was not served by a centralized municipal water supply system during the 1966 flood. In the Krasnij Farforist settlement of this region, only a minority of the population used the water supply; drinking water was taken from the river in the center of the settlement. Statistics reported by the Novgorod public health epidemiology station stated that only 40% of the people of Staraya Russa used the water supply system; 26% used the systems functioning at industrial sites, 20% used wells, 12% used river water, and 2% used artesian boreholes. This took place while in the administrative districts of the region – Staraya Russa, Novgorod, Moshinsk, Malo-Vishersk, and Chudovo – tularemia originating in bogs, lakes, and rivers was registered, the main source being water rats. The infection was spread through open reservoirs [197].

In the Moldavian SSR, the health authorities stated that the high rate of typhoid-paratyphoid infections was mainly registered in villages situated along the banks of the Dniester, downriver from the towns of Bendery and Tiraspol. These people did not receive quality drinking water; the water used was that of the Dniester River [32].

Unfavorable sanitary conditions were also behind the high rate of intestinal infections seen in Tashkent after the earthquake in 1966. The plumping and sewage systems in many buildings ceased to function. The sewage system of the city's damaged districts was badly affected [40]. According to Dubrovsky [67], 25% of Tashkent's residential houses were deprived of running water. Only 12%–15% of the people had functioning sewage services. Over 70% of industrial enterprises and institutions emptied their sewage into open reservoirs without purification. Aggravating these poor sanitary conditions was the fact that a large part of the city's population had been relocated; about 60 000 Tashkent families had to be placed in the apartments of other families and 55 000 families were put in tarpaulin tents pitched in the streets [40]. There is nothing unusual about these decisions, and such solutions are resorted to by most countries following natural disasters. What is important is to prevent a worsening of the already precarious sanitary conditions. The lessons can be taken from the 1924 Leningrad flood and the 1948 Ashkhabad earthquake.

In Uzbekistan the signs of an increase in dysentery were apparent before the earthquake which struck the republic; in the Kara-Kalpak Autonomous Republic included in the Uzbek SSR there was an outbreak of cholera in August–September 1965 [61]. According to Sharipov et al. [222], taking the 1959 dysentery index as 100%, the 1964 index was 53.1% and that for 1965 was 78.1%. After the earthquake in 1966, the incidence of dysentery and other intestinal infections in Uzbekistan increased by 1.5 as compared with the preceding years [124].

These situations are not unique to the USSR. Not long ago, only 45% of the towns in Brazil had reliable water supplies, and only 34% had sewage systems. In Chile, only 29% of towns had sewage systems [262]. And these countries are frequent victims of natural disasters.

Natural disasters of course affect medical personnel as well. The Turkmen SSR health authorities reported that as a result of the 1948 earthquake in Ashkhabad, five members of the Health Ministry central staff were killed, six injured, and five others lost. The teaching staff of the Turkmen Medical Institute comprised 114 people; 22 of these died (19.3%). Of 517 physicians employed by the republican health institutions of the Ashkhabad municipal health department, 93 died, 33 were severely injured, and four were lost; 380 remained (74.8%). Of the middle-level personnel comprising 1050 people, 135 died, 102 were injured seriously, and 36 were lost; 777 people (again 74%) survived, safe and sound [330].

On October 6–7, 1948, as a result of the considerable loss of medical personnel in Ashkhabad, only the following were availlable to provide medical aid to the injured: four professors, two senior physicians, two senior assistants, three physicians, three nurses, one hospital attendant, and 16 students. In the first 6 h after the beginning of the earthquake, only 1.7% of the physicians and 0.3% of the middle-level medical personnel of all Ashkhabad were in service.

Later on, the health authorities of the Turkmen SSR could mobilize only 50% of the regular staff of rural medical institutions to handle the lasting effects of the quake. The proportion of physicians still available in some towns of Turkmenia at January 1, 1950 was as follows: Tashauz, 36%; Chardjou, 50%; Mary, 67%. Surgical treatment was provided in only three hospitals in the 16 regions of the Chardjou district [331]. The medical personnel in the sanitary-antispidemic network of the Turkmen SSR was also reduced; only 33 of the 112.5 positions were manned at January 1, 1950.

One cannot rely on the ideal situation, in which health services' staff are always and everswhere fully manned and fully equipped. Natural disasters affect them as well. This is where the emergency medical aid service, as a mobile formation, takes on special signifance. It should always be prepared, but this is unfortunately rarely the case.

In Tashkent before the 1966 earthquakes, the emergency aid station staff was as 47.4% of capacity. Only 64.6% of vehicles were in action [77]. In the Andizhan and other adminstrative districts of the Uzbek SSR the emergency aid stations were manned at 30%–45% of capacity.

Regions prone to natural disasters must provide a sufficient number of hospital beds, and must be ready to mobilize the army reserve in an emergency. In Turkmenia in 1945, before the Ashkhabad quake, the towns had 11.7 hospital beds per 1000 people. By 1949, after the quake, this had *decreased* to 9.2 per 1000. Later on, in some places the situation was even worse. At January 1, 1950, provision with hospital beds per 1000 residents was as follows: in Nebit-Dag, 1.8; in Chardjou, 4; in Mary, 5; in Tashauz, 6.2 [332]. On average, this was a 50% decrease.

Of the 140 Tashkent medical institutions, 118 (84.3%) were damaged by the earthquake, and 5315 beds, comprising one half of the total available, were partially or totally out of service. Altogether, 1400 beds permanently available for patients with infectious diseases (80% of the total number) were out of service [40, 55]. Of 51 outpatient institutions, 37 ceased to function in buildings of their own, either temporarily or permanently [62].

No failures of the past have been taken into consideration. According to Briantzeva, Yashkov, and Nurijev [333], the number of orthopedic-traumatological beds in the Turkmen SSR in 1966 comprised only 25% of the population's actual needs (the estimate is based on the norm envisaged by the USSR Health Ministry). In Chardjou, where the 1969 flood occurred, the number of traumatological beds accounted for only 20% of those needed.

In many other countries the figures are even worse. In 1960, for example, Chile reported 4.55 hospital beds per 1000 people and Morocco 1.61; these two countries suffered catastrophic natural disasters. In Pakistan, during the night of May 12, 1965, a cyclone accompanied by a hurricane and an almost 6 m tidal wave killed 20 000 people; more than 5 million became homeless. In these conditions there was one hospital bed per 3300 people, and one physician per 7000 [89].

This is the reality pertaining to the world's public health security services. However, the problem is not only one of quantitative provision of physicians and materials. Stallones [242] seems correct in assuming that the state of the population's health ist not directly proportional to the number of physicians available. Armelagos and Katz [14], noting the health services crises in the United States, propose a reorientation from the emphasis on treatment to prophylactic activities. This obviously concerns other countries as well.

Thus, the aims of the health security authorities should be the following:

1. Provision of efficient medical first aid to the injured during the first phase of the disaster, according to vital indications
2. Treatment, evacuation, and prophylactic activities during the second phase
3. Restoration of the health network and elimination of the consequences of the disaster in the third phase

The organizational aspects of the above will be discussed in a further chapter.

To summarize, then, the following factors determine how the consequences of a natural disaster for public health can be dealt with:

1. The stress reaction; extended provision of aid serves to calm the people and to relieve stress
2. Extreme geographical conditions and location of settlements; it is important to prevent the secondary impact of the environmental factors
3. The degree to which the public health organizations are prepared for emergency situations, with a view to stabilizing the epidemic state and manifestations of illness peculiar to the area
4. The almost constant shortage of time, forces, and means in a disaster; preplanning should emphasize fast reaction and maneuverability

Medical Provision in the Initial Phase of a Natural Disaster

From the medical perspective, the sudden change in environmental conditions and mass injuries are the distinguishing factors of the initial phase of a natural disaster, which is characterized by disturbance of daily routine in general. Actually, a series of disasters follow and determine one another. Their combinded effect differs with different microregions. For many people, the burden becomes unbearable, and they become depressed over the loss of everything. It is at this stage that the largest proportion of the population in a stricken area needs medical attention within the shortest possible period of time.

Not only do the life and health of masses of people depend on efficient provision of aid; equally dependent are the further activities toward eliminating the public health consequences of the disaster and toward keeping these to a minimum. In the wider context, the authorities responsible for health services must meet the need for:

1. Medical aid to masses of people injured, evacuated, then reevacuated over a short period
2. Medical service for the population in general and for those people handling the clean-up activities
3. Restoration of the network of health institutions
4. Restoration of an epidemiologically stable environment and sanitation services

There is no problem without a potential solution. There is clearly a time gap between the moment the disaster occurs and the moment when an estimate of the situation is made and practical measures are undertaken in accordance with objective, existing capabilities. Immediately after the disaster, when it is at its most destructive, there is no time to set up efficient emergency measures or programs for restoring environmental and social equilibrium. Manpower and materials are usually insufficient, and more must be mobilized from outside. This situation is typical, and must be taken into account. The difficulties that arise can only be combatted if plans have been made for mutual aid between adjacent regions beforehand.

While a disaster is happening it is not always possible to estimate its scope, or to foresee the fast changes which may take place at new sites of damage.Therefore, it is imperative to plan, in advance, a flexible medical aid program, to be implemented as soon as a disaster begins. Such a plan would reduce apprehension in the face of the problems that arise, and these would no longer be seen as unique, unpredictable cases. The peculiarity of the situation, emotional stress, lack of experience, and the absence of reliable data for a thorough and comprehensive analysis contribute to the perception of a disaster as a tragic stroke of fate. In order to absorb it mentally and then react efficiently a certain period of time is needed.

With the arrival of emergency and medical aid teams comes the possibility of concentrating efforts and of imposing a more orderly, calm atmosphere. Only after the stress reaction has been somewhat calmed is there an opportunity to initiate extensive and intensive self-aid, and to enlist the people's cooperation with external rescue teams.

The initiative of the stricken population itself is essential for the provision of medical aid in the initial phase, because there is always a discrepancy between the available manpower and materials (in particualr, a shortage of physicians) and the needs of the people, and there are difficulties in reaching the injured, who may remain stranded for quite some time, from outside the area.

The activities of emergency teams depend on:

1. The nature of the disaster, whether it poses continuous or intermittent danger
2. The effects of extreme weather conditions (strong wind, rain, or snow, drastic changes in temperature or atmospheric pressure)
3. The extent to which communication and transportation are crippled, and the consequent isolation of the stricken area
4. The scope of evacuation, and the ensuing problem of refugees and provision of medical care to them
5. The degree to which health institutions, water supply, and sewage systems and their staff are capable of functioning

On October 6, 1948 in Ashkhabad, an earthquake damaged the emergency aid station, which could no longer function; 50% of the physicians and 28% of the nurses died. Only toward the end of the day (i.e., 12 h after the earthquake struck) did the first emergency teams from outside arrive. Altogether, during the period October 6–12, 1265 medical personnel and 48 tons of medicine and equipment were brought into the stricken area by air [135]. However, because of the lack of manpower and materials at the very beginning, the people did not receive the needed medical aid. As shown in Fig. 30, many wounded people were evacuated from the area without having received the preliminary surgical treatment necessary. As I am not in possession of reliable data concerning the nature of these wounds, I cannot estimate or analyse the complications this caused.

In natural disasters, as in war, on-the-spot provision of first aid and evacuation from the disaster zone are integral parts of the medical treatment. Surgical aid given to the injured in these two stages determines the process of medical sorting. Rescue teams and medical personnel launch their activities immediately upon arrival at the disaster site. The supplies they bring with them must enable comprehensive aid in accordance with actual needs. Rescue activities include:

a) search for and rescue of those injured and/or hidden under ruins, debris, or water;
b) administration of first aid and evacuation of the injured;
c) protection against external dangers, such as heat or cold, stray dogs, and possible infections from insects.

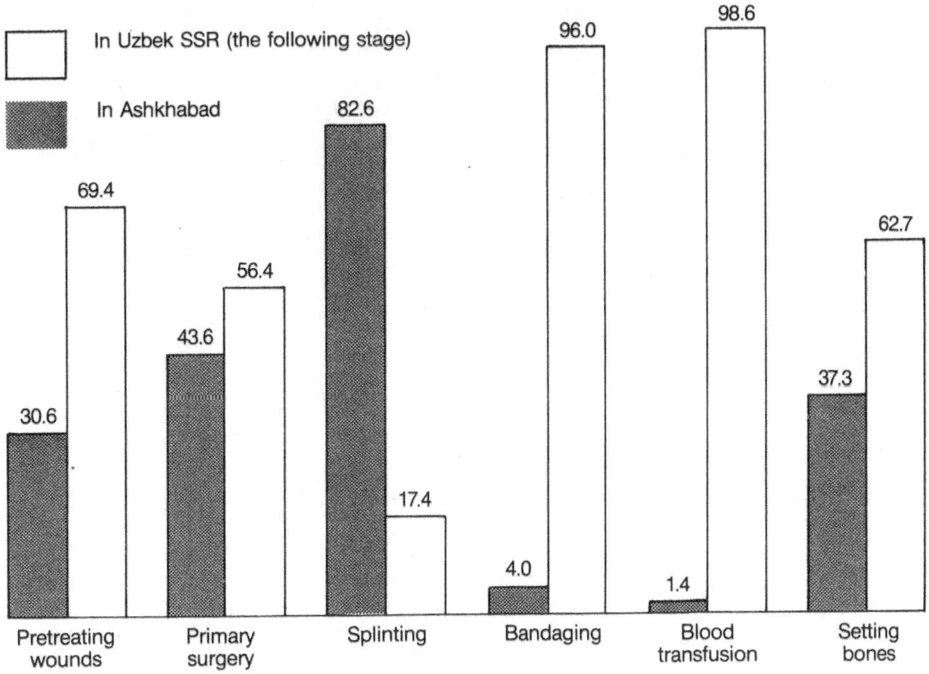

Fig. 30. Medical treatment after the Ashkhabad earthquake, 1948 (%)

In order to determine what is needed in the way of aid, it is necessary to carry out a quick medical search. This is especially important at the very beginning. A prognostic assessment can and must be made to indicate the potential sources of problems. Together with data collected from various sources, this assessment can provide an efficient prediction of the initial dynamics of the disaster and serve as a basis for the decisions which must be made. Unfortunately, the lesson of the Guatemala earthquake (1976) proves, as do so many others, that frequently such data simply do not exist. It was only on the third day after the disaster struck that the first assessment of damages was made [230]. The information collected was far from being precise, and this badly influenced the decision-making process. It took 48 h to gather medical information, including

a) the areal extent of the stricken zone,
b) the number of people affected and the gravity of injuries, and
c) the condition of health services, communications, water supply and sewage systems.

As a result of this, the coordination between emergency activities and medical aid remained insufficient. In very few countries is there a constantly functioning set of instructions and adequate storage of materials and equipment for emergency situations [17].

In most cases, initial rescue activities are improvised, and to a certain extent, this fits the actual situation and nature of the disaster, as the measures undertaken are

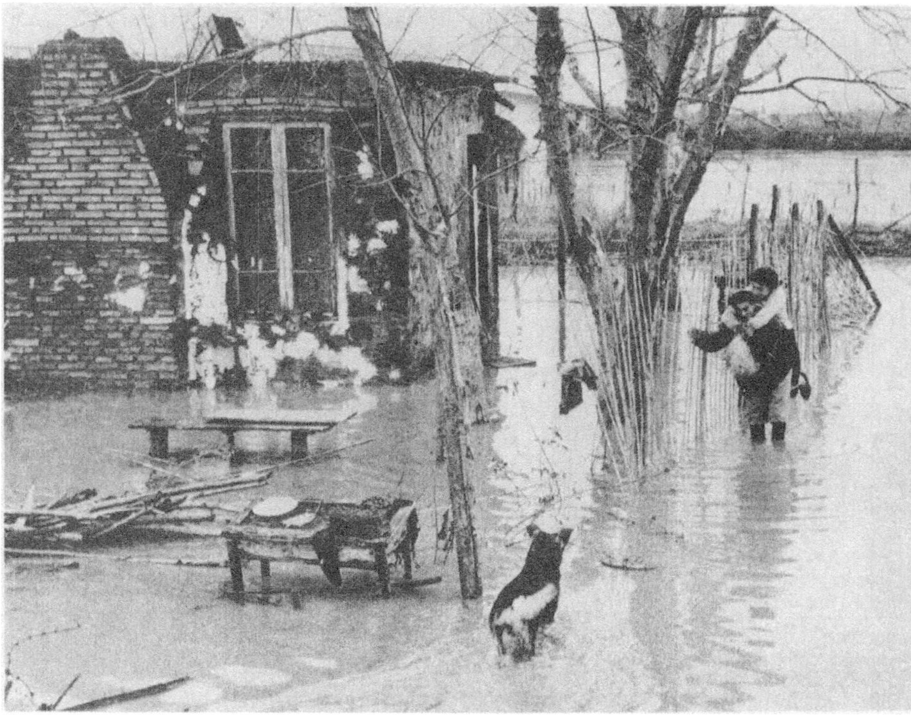

Fig. 31. Victims being carried away from the flooded zone in Fumichino, Italy, 1959 (Publiphoto)

chosen in accordance with the peculiarities of the environment and actual capabilities. In floods and tsunami people often reach safe points by swimming; from certain places the victims are rescued by hand (Fig. 31). In the Leningrad flood (Kronshtadt, 1924) women and children were carried up to 640 m; the water reached a height of 1.5 m. Emergency personnal in boats provided medical aid to people who had escaped through the windows of burning houses [335].

Efforts to reach injured people hidden under ruins entail much tension and technical difficulties (Fig. 32). Thus, rescue necessarily involves the autonomous functioning of relatively small teams, intensive physical effort, and nervous tension. Frequently, no modern machinery is available. The search for and rescue of people buried under ruins or snowslides, or those carried into the ocean by tsunami is a long and extremely arduous task. In Messina (1908), people were rescued from lower floors of buildings and from under huge layers of dust up to 12 days after the buildings crashed [336]. In Ashkhabad (1948) people waited for rescue teams under similar conditions for 10 days.

In most cases, rescue efforts are manual. It is difficult to clear away the debris of collapsed buildings; the rubble must first be broken into small pieces and can only then be removed. It is not easy to overcome the stress reaction on seeing the injured and the dead crushed under huge masses of concrete. The prolonged and intensive fight of the rescued and the rescuers under such conditions sometimes causes emotional exhaustion and emaciation. The motive driving people to continue the

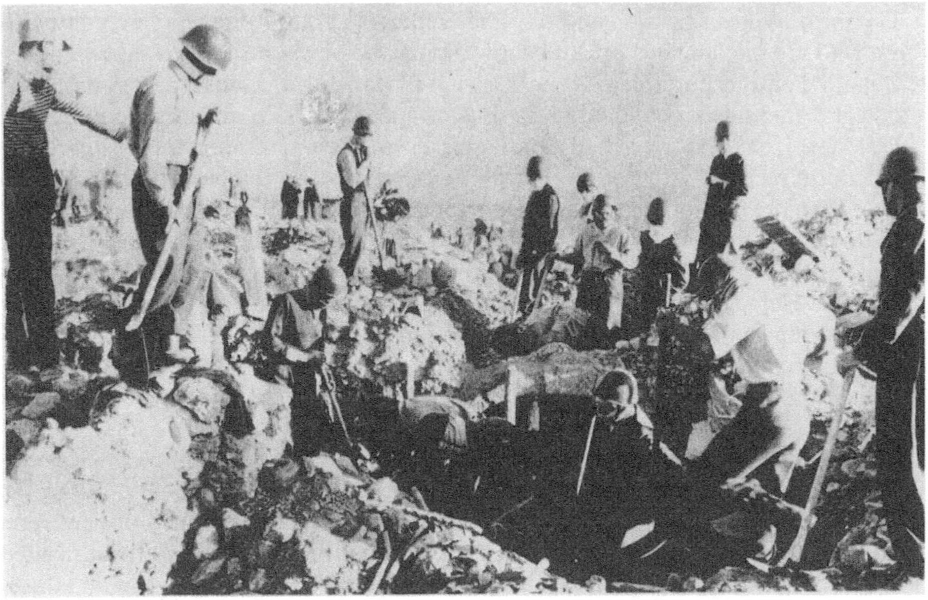

Fig. 32. Rescue works after the earthquake in Agadir, Morocco, 1960 (DPA)

fight is the profound awareness that this is the only possible chance to save lives otherwise doomed to loss under the debris.

After the effect of the initial stress reaction at the onslaught of the disaster has been overcome, attention is transferred to medical aid. People suffering from neuropsychoses under the stress reaction tend to prevail – overburdening the resources available for urgent aid to those who are truly severely injured. Medical aid is most efficient if it is given within the first 6 h following the injury; only in this period of time is it still possible to prevent the development of secondary infections [203]. For the seriously wounded, the speed with which medical treatment arrives is a question of life or death.

In light of the above facts, and considering the limited resources, an order of priorities must be determined in the provision of medical aid, and there must be a method of sorting the casualties according to the extent and nature of their injuries. People rescued from under ruins, whose extremities, thorax, and/or pelvic region may have been crushed for some hours, are in particular need of care. General and local symptoms in these cases increase during the first few hours after rescue, and death may come within 2–3 days [72] if preventive medical, antishock, and disintoxication measures are not undertaken in time. This necessitates the arrival of physicians' aid in the shortest possible time. With regard to degree of injury, the priority system, and the possibilities for medical evacuation, the injured may be classified as

a) slightly injured,
b) moderately injured, or
c) severely injured.

The third of these groups can be further subdivided into those who are conscious, those who are unconscious but still show a pulse and respiration, and those who are terminally nontransportable. A fourth group of patients are those with complicated and aggravated diseases and with diseases of undeterminded infectious etiology.

Waldner [261] has classified three phases of treatment for those injured in disasters. In phase I, whether the injured are alive or dead can be determined within minutes, before doctors are available. First aid must then be administered on the spot by people from the rescue team and its medical personnel. In phase II, aid is administered by a physician. Phase III involves the cleansing of wounds and surgical treatment. Here, as in a military operation, success depends on efficient organization. Two things in particular need to be organized:

a) evacuation of the injured from the disaster area to medical institutions, and
b) quick dispatch to the disaster area of mobile medical teams ready to provide aid at all levels required.

If there is no organization the injured are delivered to hospitals chaotically, without any plan, and in greater numbers than is sometimes necessary. Eldar [73] writes that between 12% and 40% of the population of a disaster area are delivered to hospitals. Yet the hospitals are not used rationally when they are most needed. The reception rooms are generally extremely overloaded.

According to reports of the Guatemala earthquake [230], only two of four hospitals in the system of national health services provided surgery. Twelve hours after the earthquake, all six hospitals in the country were overcrowded with the injured and the dead. Those injured in isolated mountain settlements remained without the slightest chance of receiving qualified hospital treatment.

Lack of sufficient hospital facilities in the disaster zone or nearby, causes the injured to be evacuated over long distances. In 1963 an earthquake damaged 150 settlements in the central Iranian plateau (an area of 23 000 square miles). There were no hospitals in the vicinity, and 1200 injured people had to be evacuated to Teheran, 120 miles away [73].

The absence of preorganization results in chaotic transportation of the injured to medical institutions – without preliminary surgery and without sorting. The needed treatment comes unnecessarily late. There is no universal system of providing medical aid during the initial phase of a disaster that will fit any situation and be efficient under all conditions. My own experience and research show that one of the advisable options is mobile medical groups and teams which are constantly an call, and can be dispatched immediately to the scene of the disaster. Of course, such teams must be prepared beforehand by the reponsible health authorities and institutions.

Properly equipped, the mobile medical aid group (MMAG) should include a physician (as head of the group), nurses, and corpsmen, in the ratio of 1:3:6. The medical aid they provide should include bandaging of wounds and burns; temporary arrest of bleeding; immobilization of broken extremities and damaged soft tissue; aid for those with traumatic injuries (in floods and mudslides); resuscitation for those rescued from drowning; aid for those suffering from asphyxia and frostbite (rescued from snowslides); and aid to those suffering attacks and complications of cardiovascular diseases, bronchial asthma, diabetes, mental distrubances, and other afflictions.

The nursing personnel of the MMAG should be responsible for the organization of special medical posts providing first aid to the slightly injured and those to be evacuated.

The number of such MMAGs and the area each one should service is determined by the extent of the injuries and the peculiarities of the specific disaster situation in each of the regions stricken. Following is an illustrative example. A properly equipped team, working hard for two and a half days in a totally destroyed seven-story building, was able to retrieve all those who had been under the rubble: 59% had been killed, 22% were injured, and 19% were unhurt. There may be many such buildings in a disaster zone. To estimate the personnel and materials needed, the authorities in charge of rescue activities may employ:

a) data on the size of the population of the stricken area and the number of survivors;
b) data on constructions destroyed, including the time of the occurrence;
c) the presumed nature and extent of injuries.

Appropriate communication between the rescue teams and the MMAGs ensures successful first aid activities, which are carried out until the arrival of physicians.

The appearance and course of various irreversible conditions in the severely injured are determined by the timing of qualified surgical treatment according to vital indications. Such treatment includes [258]: the arrest of external and internal bleeding and the fight against acute blood loss; complex therapy for shock and traumatic toxicosis; surgery for anaerobic infections; surgery for open pneumothorax, thoracotomy for valve pneumothorax; ventral cut in case of wounds and internal damage to the organs of the abdominal cavity, surgery for damaged urinary bladder.

To provide this treatment, and extend it if necessary, it is desirable to form mobile medical aid teams (MMATs) with these capabilities. The proportion of physicians to nursing personnel in such should be 1:3 or 1:4. The proposed functional subdivision within the MMAT is shown in Table 33. The reception department implements medical sorting according to treatment and evacuation needed. Patients are then delivered for surgery, bandaging, or general medicine, or to quarantine.

In extreme regions, the unfavorable climatic, meteorological, and communication conditions make it impossible to organize evacuation of the injured for a certain period of time. With this knowledge, the authorities should plan and implement

Table 33. Functional divisions of a mobile medical aid team

Section and function
Reception-classification
Surgery-bandaging
For slightly wounded
General medicine – isolation of:
Psychoneurological patients
Patients with known infections
Patients with suspected infections
Evacuation

a considerable extension of local hospital and evacuation departments [31, 32]. The injured and ill must be further evacuated to the nearest hospitals or by air to special medical institutions in neighboring territories.

Supplied with easily transportable equipment, an MMAT can function efficiently with the following contigent of physicians and nurses per department:

a) reception/sorting – one physician (a surgeon, heading the MMAT) and two to three nurses,
b) surgery/bandaging – three physicians and nine nurses,
c) general medicine – one or two internists and three to six nurses,
d) evacuation – one senior nurse and one assistant nurse.

Altogether, the MMAT includes five to six physicians and 16–20 nursing personnel. Additional resources would include a drug dispensary, X-ray appliances, a laboratory, and possibly an administrative unit with a kitchen.

As stated above, extreme regional conditions may cause a delay in the evacuation of people in general and/or of patients being treated by the MMAT. To prevent complications there must be specialized on-site medical aid. The scope of such medical provision can be seen in Table 34, compiled from material on 11 108 cases of injuries in the 1948 Ashkhabad earthquake [336] and the report of the German field hospital which functioned in Peru from May 10 to July 27 after the 1970 earthquake [93].

There may be a need for the following types of specialized medical aid: surgery facilities for ophthalmology, orthopedics, traumatology and gynecology; therapeutic; psychiatry; pediatrics. It is therefore wise to include in the MMAT one or two additional physicians and two or four additional nurses, as well as the necessary

Table 34. Injuries and diseases resulting from Ashkhabad earthquake (1948) and Peru earthquake (1970)

	%
Ashkhabad earthquake (1948)[a]	
Wounded[b]	50.0
Internal diseases	11.7
Eye diseases and injuries	11.0
Children's diseases	6.8
Gynecological disorders	4.6
Other	15.9
Peru earthquake (1970)	
Respiratory diseases	24.0
Nervous	19.0
Cases for surgery	13.0
Digestiv disorders	12.0
Urogenital disorders	8.0
Rheumatic diseases	6.0
Cardiac and circulatory diseases	5.0
Other	13.0

[a] Based on 11 108 cases
[b] Severely wounded, needing evacuation, 20.2%; slightly to moderately wounded, 79.8%

equipment. The MMAT with specialized brigades constitutes a qualitatively new type of team, the extended one. This extended mobile medical aid team (EMMAT) can provide qualified specialized treatment, including reanimation and prophylaxis for the post-reanimation pathology of the brain. This is necessary for three reasons [5]:

a) continuous artificial ventilation of the lungs, or auxiliary ventilation after restoration of blood circulation,
b) the fight against post-reanimation complications; and
c) protection of the brain from hypoxia, as well as a more comprehensive and quicker restoration of its functions.

During the inital phase of a natural disaster there is a particular need for intensive antiepidemiological measures, especially to protect children, against intestinal and other infections. This is all the more important if the sanitary situation prior to the disaster was unsatisfactory, or if the area has a history of epidemics. The EMMAT must consider including in its framework a mobile antiepidemic team (MAET) to cover this need. The MAET should consist of two or three physicians (an epidemiologist, an expert in local domestic hygiene, and a bacteriologist) and five to six nurses.

The MAET must be capable of and equipped for organizing an on-site laboratory and of launching antiepidemic and disinfective activities including defining standards for observation an quarantine; organizing an antiepidemic regime, if necessary, in the evacuation lines and at evacuation points; organizing nutrition control and water supply control – a matter of the utmost importance.

Evacuation is an integral part of medical aid to the injured, who are taken to hospitals and other medical institutions capable of providing treatment to the extent needed. Evacuees can amount to a considerable proportion of the population. In the Ashkhabad earthquake, 69.5% of the severely injured were evacuated. They were sent to towns of the Uzbek SSR (35.8%), the Azerbaijan SSR (33.7%), and to other towns of the Turkmen SSR itself (30.5%). According to Vishnevsky's report [337], of those evacuated to the Uzbek SSR, 51.2% were women, 36.1% men, and 12.7% children. This correponds to the structure of the injuries in this disaster in general, women and children constituting the main part of the population injured.

The evacuation procedure depends on the rescue activities undertaken, the organization of medical aid, and the communication conditions at the time in question. Evacuation after the Ashkhabad earthquake was essentially completed within the first 4 days (83.9%). This was the period of broad-scale rescue work and intensive medical care provided by teams which had arrived in the stricken zone, properly equipped.

The principal means of evacuation was air transport (79.6%) shown in Fig. 33 [32]; 240 planes were used in the air bridge, 120 of them transporting injured daily [338]. An efficient air bridge makes it possible to bring in manpower and materials quickly and to take out the injured who have been prepared for evacuation.

Figure 34 illustrates a part of a disaster zone in which the following resources are available:

1. Rescue team, sanitary divisions of civil defense teams, and volunteers giving first aid

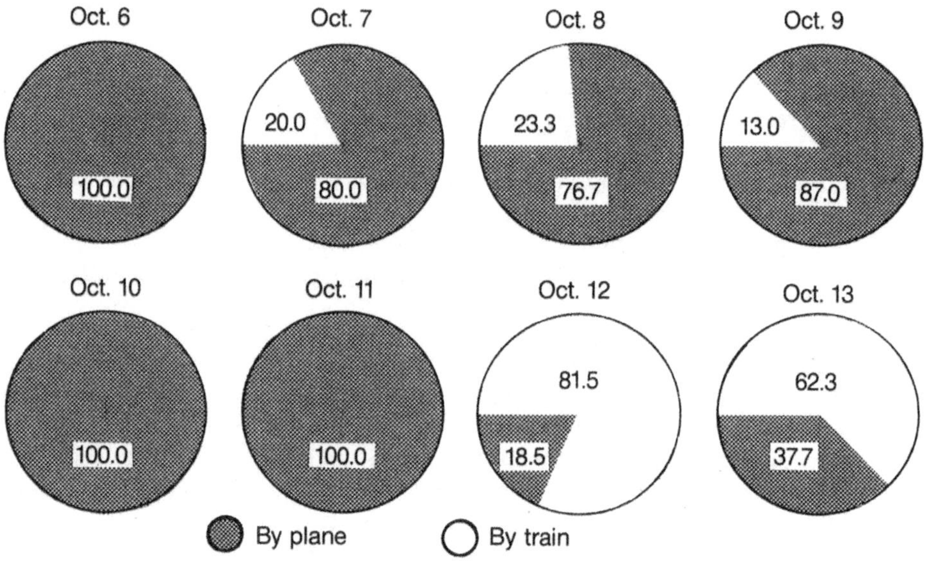

Fig. 33. Evacuation of injured from Ashkhabad according to type of transport (%). Numbers above diagrams indicate dates (earthquake took place on October 5, 1948) [32]

2. MMAGs organizing transport to medical posts where first aid and treatment by physicians will be provided (according to vital indications)
3. MMATs providing treatment by physicians and qualified surgeons (according to vital indications)
4. EMMATs following regular MMATs and providing specialized, qualified aid
5. MAETs providing antiepidemic measures
6. Evacuation points where people are gathered for further evacuation and are given medical care if needed

The scheme in Fig. 34 specifies the transportation for injured and other patients carried on stretchers. If conditons are such that communication and transportation are readily available, emergency measures and medical aid should be coordinated on a overall scale, covering the entire disaster area. This should be done by the staff including medical specialists for emergency activities control. Activities in particular sections of the disaster area should be coordinated by the commanders of rescue and medical teams.

The health services should have the power to provide the necessary manpower and materials. Implementation of recommendations drawn from such a system entails coorperation between the medical services or the civil defense system, military medical services, and public and private medical institutions. Such cooperation would enable the creation of reserve forces to form medical teams in an emergency situation. In many countries, however, there is no possibility of such efficient cooperation. This is especially true of small and/or poor countries, where the general health services system has not yet been developed properly. What makes

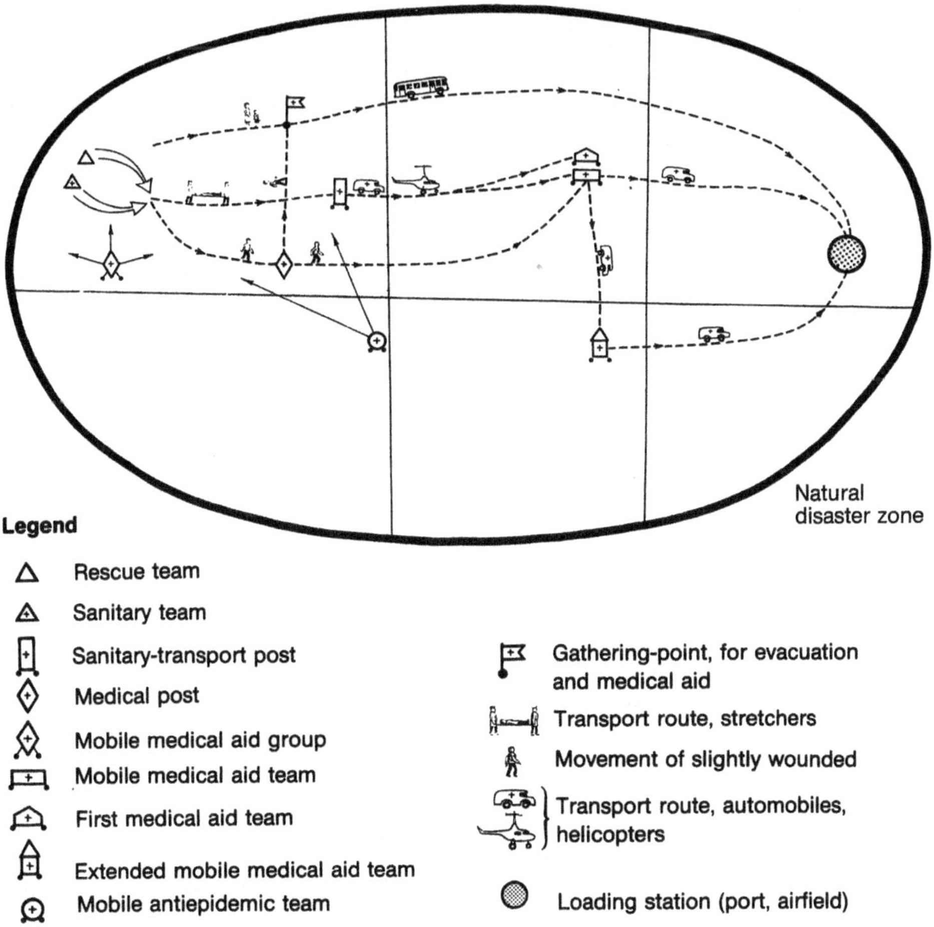

Fig. 34. Organization of medical aid in the natural disaster zone (starting period)

the situation even more difficult is lack of centralization of these services and of centralized delegation of responsibilities. Thus, many institutions face tremendous difficulties when requird to assign their forces to the combined efforts of providing medical aid to the victims of a natural disaster. The same problems are faced in organizing the small teams described above. For all that, the sometimes hidden potential and existing possibilities in any country are rarely used efficiently, the main reason frequently being lack of an organizational basis.

The experience of the earthquake [230] showed how diffuse and uncoordinated are the sources providing medical personnel and equipement in Guatemala, as well as in other countries which expressed their readiness to help. Some of the equipment desperately needed was at the disposal of the American embassy and in warehouses owned by Panama. Contributions came from various voluntary agencies and Guatemalan merchants. Tremendous effort was expended to solve the transportation problems, and to overcome the difficulties with storage facilities (refrigerators) for medicines. Foreign volunteers arrived in Guatemala without equipment or instructions. Many of them had no idea of the conditions awaiting them in the disaster zone. The language barrier obstructed contact with the people they were to help.

To avoid such chaos, a variant of a system is recommended to provide reserve medical forces and means in the event of natural disaster. This system envisages the organizaion of special complex brigades prepared in advance, including physicians, nurses, and junior personnel, appropriately equipped on the basis of existing medical institutions. I have organized such brigades [30, 31, 32] which included relevant specialists (internists, surgeons, roentgenologists and others). Because of their background and the appliances at their disposal, they were capable of develping on-the-spot MMAGs and the MMAT and EMMAT.

Such cooperation of medical forces situated in the disaster area and nearby is important [30, 31, 32]. The experience of the Tashkent earthquake (1966) shows that any other form of medical aid provision is inefficient. A large group of physicians, nurses, and specialists (160 people) arrived from Moscow and was dispersed throughout Tashkent, filling staff vacancies and giving medical treatment not connected with the earthquake and even irrelevant to their specialities and organizational backgrounds.

Holloway [113] has noted the necessity of supplying each town and region with a plan for using existing local medical resources under conditions of a natural disaster. This must be done in consideration of eventual cooperation with forces arriving from outside. This would provide maneuverability in the critical and unexpected circumstances caused by the malfunctioning of medical institutions and others.

We have considered the problems involved with a system of mobile medical forces and materials and their tasks during the initial period of a natural disaster. The scheme suggested cannot be universally applied, but is presented as a basis, open to correction and modification in light of actual conditions.

In the next stage of the period directly following a disaster, the measures undertaken to eliminate the public health consequences are dependent upon whether or not the injurious effects continue; upon medicogeographical conditions; upon the availability of reserve forces and material and their maneuverability; and upon the state of development of local health services and their preparedness to act in the extreme situation of mass injuries and destruction. The success of such activities is determined by a correct assessment of the situation and the speed with which they are performed. Table 35 presents a scheme for a health services system for dealing with the public health consequences of natural disasters. It concretizes the two aspects of the plan that directly concern the health authorities. The first is provision of medical aid proper and the evacuation of the injured, and the second is the implementation of prophylactic sanitary measures as comprehensively as possible.

Table 35. Elimination of public health consequences of natural disasters

Main determining factors	Activities	Forces and means
Character, scope, and duration of disaster	Assessment of consequences, implementation of rescue/aid plan worked out beforehand	Centrally coordinated emergency medical team
Extreme conditions: a) natural factors, e.g., mountainous area, atmospheric precipitation, drastic temperature changes, etc.; b) destruction of health service system, water supply, sewage, residential buildings, municipal, domestic institutions	Comprehensive medical aid to: injured; evacuated/reevacuated, refugees; rescue personnel	External mobile medical teams: health institutions, public and private medical institutions (in co-operation); military medical services, medical services of civil defense organizations
Socioeconomic chaos (with hunger), underlying all epidemic processes directly following calamity	Treatment and prophylaxis of: a) acute and complicated neuropsychological, cardiovascular diseases, diabetes, bronchial asthma, and others; b) children's intestinal infectious diseases; c) effects of overcooling or overheating; d) diseases caused by bites of dogs or insects (rabies, leishmaniasis, malaria, parasitic typhoid Restoration of public health service system and promotion of its further development	Extant and restored public health institutions

Of the utmost importance for the elimination of the public health consequences is appropriate and adequate materials:

1. The data I proposed for the compilation of nosoprognostic maps, specifying potential natural disasters in any given territory
2. A general description of the disaster once it has occurred, and information on the extent of damaged and injuries caused
3. Constantly updated facts on the public health consequences, the environmental conditions as affected by the disaster, and the procedures being followed for their elimination

After the problems caused by such disaster have been eliminated, the new experience must be thoroughly analyzed and considered as a lesson for the future.

Medical Provision During Evacuation After a Natural Disaster

In the complex of protective measures against a natural disaster, evacuation occupies an important place [125]. This problem appears to be insufficiently covered in the literature, especially with regard to its medical aspects.

Lack of preparedness to implement evacuation has frequently been observed. The earthquake and tsunami of September 1, 1923 caught the Japanese government unawares; it was only on the second day of the disaster that they began with evacuation. A tsunami struck the Kuril Islands on November 4–5, 1952. No evacuation at all took place before the disaster because there was no warning services to warn of the tsunami's approach, and general ignorance of the features of such a phenomenon.

People leave their homes unwillingly, and overcoming their negative reaction to warnings calling for evacuation, is often a great problem. In some cases there is lack of concern, in others a tendency to take risks, as people cannot imagine or foresee the gravity of the consequences.

The general atmosphere in a disaster, as it reaches the critical points, speaks for the fact that much time has been wasted and preventive measures not taken. Honolulu was warned twice (1958, 1959) of oncoming tsunami. People did not believe the warnings and no evacuation was begun [214]. According to Lachman, Tatsuoka, and Bank [147], the signal warning of the approaching wave lasted for 20 m in the city of Hilo (Hawaii Island), more than 4 h before it hit. Ninety-five percent of the people heard the signal but only 41% left for safer places. Of those who heard the signal and stayed, 6% said they did not know what it meant, and 4.3% said they had stayed on the coast to observe the "picturesque scene".

The Novgorod (USSR) flood began on April 1, 1966. It reached its apogee in the town of Novgorod proper on May 13 (at 765 cm above the usual level) and in Staraya Russa on May 12 (at 611 cm above normal). The flood ended in the middle of July. In Staraya Russa, where 41.3% of the streets were totally flooded and 28.8% partially (Fig. 35), only 3000 families were evacuated. Those who refused evacuation lived in the garrets of their houses. There was an absence of reliable prognostic information, and many preferred to temporize. Such a "solution" can necessitate implementation of evacuation exactly during the period of the disaster's strongest effects, under critical conditions.

In Voroshilovgrad (USSR) on March 26, 1964, i.e., 6 days after a flood had begun, the situation reached its critical apex. On that day, 57.5% of all evacuations took place [32]. Such a situation causes especially high expenses.

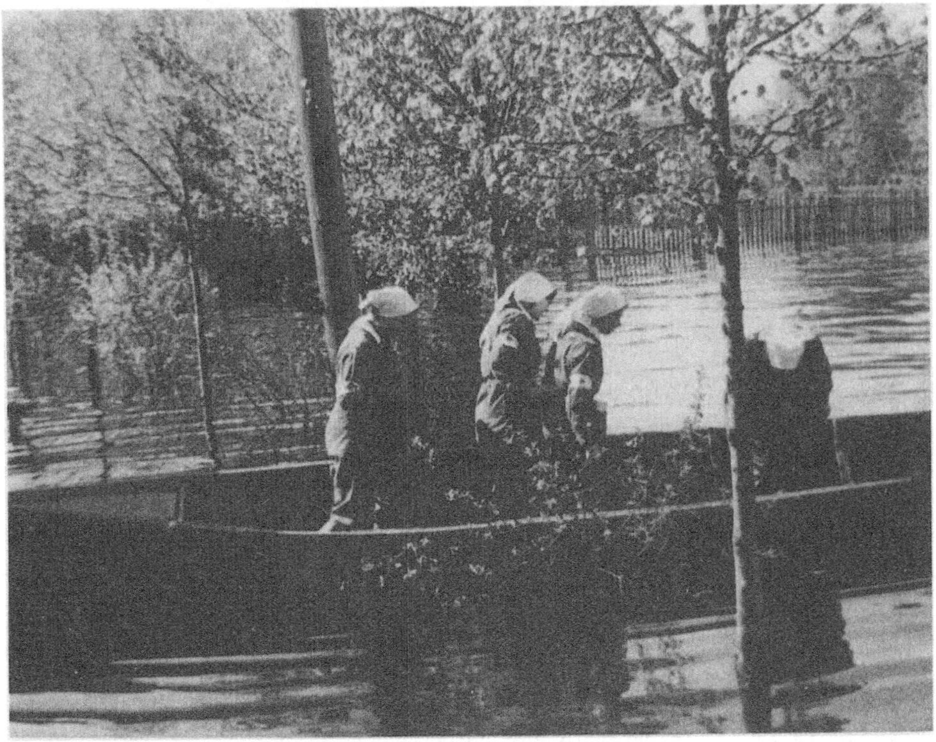

Fig. 35. Flooded part of the town of Staraya Russa, May 1966 [32]

Implementation of evacuation can become an impossible task if the communication and transportation facilities are put out of use. Night aggravates the situation. Storms and strong, force-12 winds in the night of February 16, 1962 caused a huge sea wave to hit the North Sea coast. Several dikes were broken through, and an area covering 150 km^2 (Federal Republic of Germany) was flooded. There were 307 people killed and 40 000 reported homeless. Damages were estimated at DM 1 billion. The bulk of the rescue activities were carried out by 40 000 members of the Bundeswehr. Red Cross units were active in providing evacuation help and medical aid. It is worthy of note that helicopters were most useful; 1117 people were rescued with them.

Practical evacuation depends on the people's attitude, the continuing effects of the disaster, especially at night, and the availability of the necessary manpower and means capable of performing under the particular conditions of the disaster in question. This concerns transportation especially – air (helicopters and planes), water (boats, cutters, river and sea ships), and land vehicles capable of driving over rough terrain.

Timely evacuation prevents chaotic and disorderly migration of refugees, minimizes human losses, and facilitates the restoration of sanitation and good public health conditions. Without a thorough evacuation plan complications ensue, especially for public health. The relocation of masses of people under drastically changed ecological conditions brings about outbreaks of epidemics [7]. Unfavorable weather conditions and the continuation of a raging hurricane or a flood often lead to malfunctioning or breakdown of the transportation and communication networks. Such factors as mountain relief, narrow streets, the outbreak of fires, and blocked roads cause delays in evacuation. Especially dangerous are cities with particular features of location, such as San Francisco and Petropavlovsk-Kamchatsk.

Plans for emergency must be put into action immediately upon assessment of the coming danger and its possible consequences. Since evacuation is normally handled within a country's borders, we are talking about internal migration. Ravenstein [207] distinguishes between local, short-distance, long-distance, and "stage" migrants.

Evacuation is closely connected with the nature and extent of the effects of a disaster. In this respect, natural disasters can be subdivided as follows:

1. According to timing and the possibility of determining their appearance
   a) Suddenly appearing, within an hour or two, where prediction is difficult to impossible, and the time for implementation of plans for protection and rescue is very limited
   b) Gradually appearing, over several days or weeks, where prediction is more or less precise, and time is relatively sufficient for implementation of plans
2. According to extent of damage and territory involved
   a) Limited to one or several settlements, with no need for evacuation
   b) On a large scale, covering an extended region or a large part of a country, and necessitating mass evacuation
3. According to duration of the effects of the disaster
   a) Short-term (1–2 days), with short-term evacuation on the population
   b) Long-term (up to 2 months and more), with long-term evacuation

In the group of natural disasters which can be predicted with a certain degree of exactness (typhoons, floods due to heavy rains and fast-melting snow, meteorological tsunami) the time available for evacuation may be an hour, several hours, or a day and more. In the group of suddenly appearing disasters for which it is difficult or practically impossible to issue warnings (earthquakes, tsunami caused by underwater volcanic eruptions, floods caused by dam breaks) evacuation activities can at best coincide with the effects of the disaster, and are often only carried out afterwards. In either of the two types of disasters, safe places for evacuation can be situated

a) near the affected zone (e.g., coastal heights in tsunami), or
b) far from the affected zone (especially in large-scale earthquakes or floods).

The evacuated are frequently relocated within the municipal borders of the stricken area. In the USSR people are generally placed in public buildings and schools, in tents specially put up for this purpose, or in the apartments of people living in safe areas, thus increasing the population density of these residential areas.

The following must be considered in planning for evacuation:

a) the time of day and the season of the year,
b) geographical conditions and geographical pathology of the stricken zone,
c) the state of communications and transportation, employment conditions, and normal domestic conditions.

The time needed for evacuation depends on the given geographical and communication conditions; in some cases only a day is needed to deliver the evacuated to safe places, while in others it may take much longer. It is not always possible to determine this time beforehand.

Most of the evacuation is completed within the first few days following a disaster. This is the periods in which rescue activities are launched on a full scale and maximum medical aid is provided. After the Ashkhabad earthquake, 83.9% of the injured and ill were evacuated in the first 4 days [32]. Since the railway network was no longer functioning, 79.6% of them were carried by air [32]. Organized air bridges enable fast delivery of rescue teams and materials to the disaster area and – as return cargo – evacuation of the injured to places especially prepared for them. This was the experience after the earthquake at Skopje, Yugoslavia in 1963.

Practical organization of evacuation requires differentiating between the contingents of the evacuated and setting priorities. In any case, of primary importance is the evacuation of those people who cannot participate in any further protection/rescue activities. These are: preschool and school children, their mothers and others assigned to care for them (Fig. 36); pregnant women; the aged; the ill – both those being treated in hospitals and those at home; and invalids.

In Canada there is a priority system for determining the evacuation order in hospitals under emergency conditions. Patients are divided into four groups:

1. Those under observation after surgical interference are discharged and transferred to ambulatory treatment with follow-up medical observation

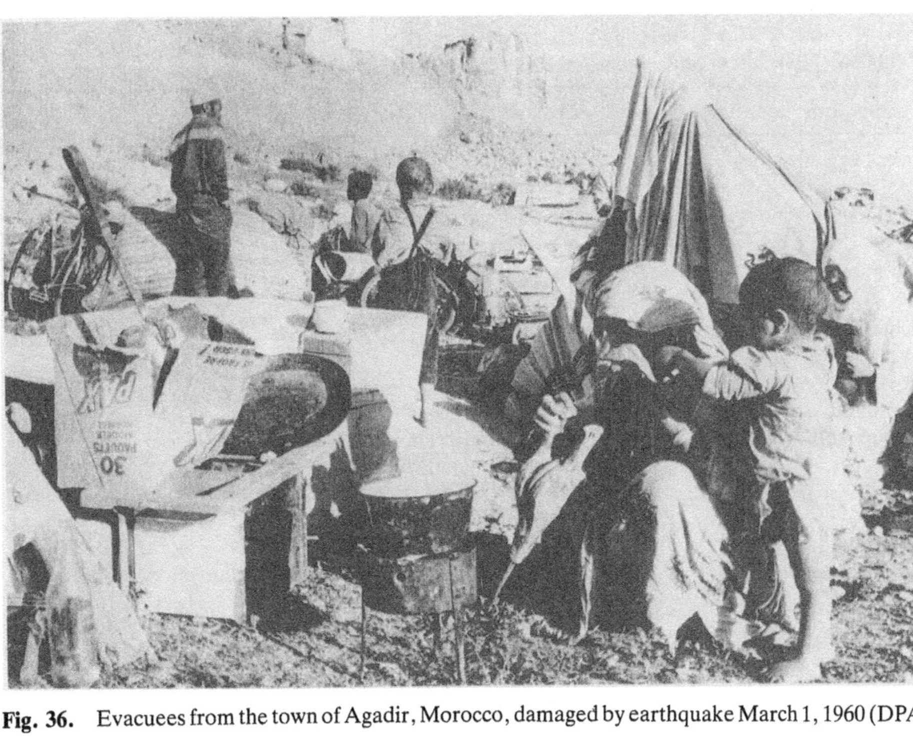

Fig. 36. Evacuees from the town of Agadir, Morocco, damaged by earthquake March 1, 1960 (DPA)

2. Those needing medical care, bandaging, and other medical or paramedical procedures are also discharged and assigned to further observation and treatment by intermediate-level medical personnel
3. Postoperational and critically ill patients who need transportation on stretchers are evacuated next. These may comprise 20%–25% of the total number of patients in the hospital
4. Nontransportable patients remain in the hospital with medical personnel who stay behind specifically to treat them – all of them under a certain amount of risk

The stages of evacuating are the establishment of gathering points for evacuees, the arrival of the evacuees at the assigned destination, the settling of the evacuees. Each stage has its particular characteristics. Table 36 offers a schematic consideration of the elements of implementation and provision at each one, and a classification of evacuation activities as determined bay the type of disaster. The classification helps in the organization of provision of medical aid to the evacuees and in the planning of measures indispensable at each of the specified stages.

In the USSR, the gathering points for evacuees are set up at places of work, in educational institutions, and in housing management offices. Each point accommodates 2000–2500 people and includes a medical dispensary with a physician and a nurse.

The evacuees are transported by automobile columns, each comprised of 20–30 vehicles. Land-route columns for those evacuated on foot are planned for the movement of 100–150 people. To provide medical care en route, MMAGs should be organized, consisting of one physician, two or three nurses, and up to six medical

Table 36. Evacuation after a natural disaster

Factors to be considered	Possibilities
Initial organization	Sudden Preliminary
Destination	Nearest safe neighborhood Far away
Duration	Short term (a few days) Long term (more than a month, up to a year and more)
Time/season	Daytime Nighttime Summer Autumn–winter and spring
Groups to be evacuated	Entire population Mostly women, children, and elderly Diseased, those needing transportation under a) special conditions, and b) regular conditions
Special considerations	Geographic peculiarities (cold/hot climate, mountains, etc.) Geographic pathology Labour conditions and everyday domestic conditions Communications conditions Mass movement of refugees (witnessing large-scale disorder and lack of organization)

attendants, all properly equipped. MMAGs should be placed at crossroads, river crossings, mountain passes, and other places of possible concentration of the evacuees [32]. Taking into account meteorological, climatic, an other possibly unfavorable conditions, planners must envisage the necessity of providing hot-food preparation at these points, blankets and warm clothing, observation and quarantine facilities.

To provide medical aid to the evacuees moving along highways, organization of first aid posts seems advisable. These could consist of one nurse and two medical attendants.

In countries with a highly developed railway network, trains will be the most efficient means of transferring the people to safe places. One physician and one nurse should be assigned for each train carrying more than 1000 people [32]. Long-distance trains must include a quarantine wagon.

The use of health control posts (HCP) in the USSR during the Second World War merits attenion. The HCP included the following personnel: head of the post (physician), four nurses, two sanitary workers (responsible for disinfection activities). The functions of the HCP were to identify those with infections and fevers at the railway stations and in the trains, and to organize sanitary treatment in the trains and disinfection of the wagons. The fact that evacuees congregate and are detained at large railway stations and major junctions makes it desirable to send complex mobile brigades of physicians and nurses with necessary equipment there. Evacuation by rail, or any other kind of transport under unsatisfactory sanitary-epidemiological conditions, is fraught with possibilities for the spread of infections. Therefore, detection and isolation of the diseased and further antiepidemic measures are of special significance. Disinfection detachments with quarantine and laboratory wagons should be organized for this purpose.

Provision of food and other services to the evacuees who have been placed under observation and in quarantine must be the responsibility of the observation posts. Thus, flexible provision of medical care to the evacuees involves various organizations acting in cooperation, and functionally succeeding each other.

Where evacuation is by sea or river transportation, medical aid is provided at posts set up on ships at the landing piers, or on floating medical facilities. From the point of view of speed, of course, evacuation by air is the most efficient. In this case, medical aid must be organized in neighborhoods closest to airports, on landing strips, and at suitable landing spots for helicopters. For any number of reasons there may be temporary delays in evacuation, and for such a situation it is necessary to provide reinforcement of the medical posts providing health services at the sites where the people are collected and waiting to be evacuated.

The nature of a disaster's effects can make it necessary to evacuate people by road within the municipal borders of the city stricken. This can lead to an increase in road traffic accidents and injuries. This pertains especially to mountainous areas. An instructive example is San Francisco, where the relatively narrow streets are full of sharp ascents and descents. Another aggravating factor is the outbreak of fires, especially in congested areas.

In the Tashkent earthquake in 1966, those evacuated within the city's borders were placed in 29 tent camps served by medical posts. Each camp of 160 tents was provided with a medical post, which had one medical assistant, five nurses, and four sanitary attendants. This personnel provided a 24 h watch. The Deputy Health Minister of the Uzbek SSR, V. M. Boiko, stated that in many of the camps the basic sanitary-hygienic requirements were violated [339]. Together with other reasons, this created an unsatisfactory epidemiological situation, particularly with regard to gastrointestinal infections.

Epidemic conditions are determined by

a) a worsening of the sanitary situation as a result of damages caused by the disaster and the forced migration of a considerable part of the population;
b) the emergency atmosphere, which functions as a stress factor, lowering the physical and mental stability and the immunobiological reactivity of people, and making them more susceptible to diseases;
c) worsening nutrition, domestic conditions, and medical care.

In light of the above, data concerning morbidity and mortality among the evacuees in the USSR during the Second World War are of interest. Korsunskaya [139] reported that in large cities in the USSR there was a sharp increase in measles and whooping cough, especially among the evacuated. In Cheliabinsk, 20% of scarlet fever patients and 24% of diphtheria patients were evacuated children. A higher evacuee mortality is shown by data reflecting the situation in the Kazakh SSR, where the evacuated comprised 42.1% of those who died in November 1941 in the Djambul region, 33.1% in the South Kazakhstan region, and 19.1% in Alma-Ata [340]. For the first quarter of 1942 in the city of Alma-Ata itself, of 930 patients with epidemic typhus, 737 (79.2%) had arrived on trains, and only 193 (20.8%) were local residents [341].

The situation following a natural disaster may be similar. Organization of medical care for the stricken population at all stages of its evacuation requires special attention. First aid constitutes the basis of medical aid, because forces and means are limited, and the number of those to be served is great. Initial medical assistance is either self-administered or rendered by fellow victims. Rescue teams then take over, carrying out the following measures [32]: implementation of the basic, indispensable transportation, and delivery of medicine to those suffering from cardiovascular diseases, lung diseases, diabetes, etc.; bandaging of injuries and burns; temporary arrest of bleeding; immobilization of broken limbs and damaged soft tissue; administration of aid in cases of overcooling or overheating, and to those rescued from drowning. An important role in the system of first aid is played by the intermediate-level medical personnel, who are responsible for checking and correcting bandages and tourniquets and for administrating analgesics and cardiac medicine.

Among the evacuated will be a contingent of chronic patients suffering aggravations and needing treatment by doctors. The situation in the initial phase of a disaster enables only treatment according to vital indications and to the extent of available medical facilities. This covers identification of the injured and diseased, and providing first the aid of a physician according to vital indications, then sending those in need of further treatment to the appropriate medical institution; fighting bleeding, implementing antishock measures, and giving aid to those rescued from drowning; rehabilitation of disturbed cardiac and respiratory functions, prevention of and fighting against pulmonary edema (especially in high-altitude conditions) and asphyxia; dealing with overcooling, frostbite, and overheating; bandaging of injuries, or correction of previous bandages; immobilization of broken extremities and extensively damaged soft tissue; hospitalization of nontransportable patients and provision of treatment.

Such medical aid is frequently provided while evacuees are literally in motion, on their way to safer places, as well as on their arrival at the destination or temporary shelter. Most refugees have no means with which to take care of their own needs, and aid must come from outside.

Unsanitary conditions caused by the movement of refugees can be prevented by eliminating the reasons for evacuation as a result of a natural disaster, or by organizing the evacuation and provision of medical aid ahead of time. A schematic outline of provision of medical aid to a population evacuated in an emergency

Table 37. Medical aid given to population evacuated because of natural disaster

Level of medical help	Stage of evacuation	Aid administered by	Provision of aid in accordance with character of evacuation			
			Sudden	Preliminary	Short term, near zone of calamity	Long term, for from zone of calamity
First aid	Starting period	Population itself (self-aid, mutual aid); rescue teams; medical post at gathering point	+	+	+	+
Paramedical aid	Gathering point	Medical post at gathering point; mobile medical teams (MMAT)	–	+	+	+
	En route	MMAT, paramedical personnel accompanying trains	+	+	+	+
	Place of arrival	Medical post at receiving point	+	+	+	+
Treatment by doctors	Gathering point	Medical post at gathering point	–	+	+	+
	En route	MMAT, physicians accompanying trains	+	+	+	+
	Place of arrival	Medical post at receiving point	+	+	+	+
Qualified and specialized medical aid	Gathering point	–	–	–	–	–
	En route	–	–	–	–	–
	Place of arrival	Medical post at receiving point through to hospitals of local health service system	+	+	+ according to vital indications	+
Anti-epidemic provision	Gathering point	Medical post at gathering point	–	+	+ (according to epidemiological indications)	+
	En route	Accompanying medical personnel	+	+	+ (according to epidemiological indications)	+
	Place of arrival	Medical post at receiving point	+	+	+ (according to epidemiological indications)	+

situation is presented in Table 37. Its aim is timely planning of provision of medical aid to the evacuated population at the different stages of the evacuation.

Along with the elimination of the consequences of a natural disaster is the process of reevacuation. Observing priorities in reevacuating particular contingents of the previously evacuated population, and providing appropriate medical care, will help prevent a worsening of the public health situation. To this purpose there must be selective and general examinations to identify individuals with or those suspected of having infections, and to detain them from reevacuation. The reevacuated must receive hygienic care, and those with definite or suspected infections must be committed to hospitals.

Upon arrival at their destinations, the reevacuated – as well as contingents of the indigenous population – may find themselves in the difficult situation of having insufficient medical care. In Ashkhabad, for 7 months from November 1948 until May 1949, the medical network was situated in tents. By November 1949, 1500 beds were again in service, but any specialized treatment still had to be provided in other Soviet republics [342].

When order has been reestablished and reevacuation accomplished, the functions of the medical institutions are determined by the structure of morbidity. This depends on the effects of the disaster, especially as manifested during short-term evacuation, and the environmental conditions. The report of the Voroshilovgrad hospital no. 4 polyclinic (which served the population of the flooded Kamenebrodsky district in 1964) illustrates this (Table 38). The greatest increases in patients' visits to the polyclinic were registered for those with traumas (92.7%), urinary diseases (29%), curable diseases (27.2%), and ear-nose-throat diseases (25.5%). A decrease in visits was noticed in the following departments: ophthalmology, neurology, dermatology, surgery, and oncology. This is explained by the fact that during the flood, some physicians could not provide a full range of treatment in unadapted quarters. Thus, the decrease in patients' visits to these departments does not necessarily reflect a decrease in patients' need for these services.

Disturbances in the normal functioning of the hospital brought about changes in the indices regarding the occupation of beds. According to the plan, the annual number of occupied days per bed in 1964 was supposed to be 334.7; in fact, it was

Table 38. Voroshilovgrad Municipal Hospital No. 4, Polyclinic. Breakdown of patients for 1964 in comparison with previous year (1963 = 100%)

	Increase (%)	Decrease (%)
Traumatology	92.7	
Urology	29.0	
General medicine	27.2	
Ear, nose, throat	25.5	
Obstetrics-gynecology	19.2	
Endocrinology	18.2	
Ophthalmology		1.0
Neurology		2.0
Dermatology		5.9
Surgery		21.0
Oncology		42.7

278.4 (82.3% of the target [343]). As part of the organization of the system of medical institutions during the period of elimination of the consequences of a disaster, this index must be kept under control.

Nonorganized, and consequently unprovided-for return of the evacuated can mean a worsening of the sanitary-epidemiological situation. The connection between reevacuation and the high measles morbidity in Leningrad during the Second World War [344] and the increase in epidemic typhus, especially at the Dno, Malaya Vishera, Novgorod, and other railway stations [345] serve as instructive examples. And upon reevacuation of the children to Moscow in 1943, the index of diphtheria cases increased considerably [346].

This leads to the following conclusions:

1. Evacuation occupies an important place in the system of protection and aid following a natural disaster; properly carried out, it can reduce the severity of the public health consequences
2. The basic medical care provided to evacuees is first aid and the care of the first physician, according to vital indications
3. The groups formed to administer medical aid to the evacuated must be flexible, maneuverable, and capable of envisaging the integrity and succession of activities at the different stages of evacuation. It appears justifiable to organize medical posts at evacuation points, MMAGs, HCPs, observation posts, and other both mobile and stationary sanitary-medical units
4. Public health measures take on a special significance when reevacuation has been completed and order restored

Evacuees and refugees are vulnerable to a variety of mental symptoms because of separation from their families, loss of relatives, and their material losses. Among Second World War refugees in Norway, the frequency of reactive psychosis reached 2.29%, with paranoia especially common [71]. Ecological pessimism has acquired a vast following in the modern world, and the psychosis of "how to survive if something happens" will obviously exert a negative effect upon the general mood. Depression will be aggravated. Timely and orderly evacuation and well-planned relocation of the population can calm the atmosphere and prevent aggravation of mental and emotional disturbances. This depends on the attitudes of the relevant state organs and institutions, the evacuees themselves, and the population in the surrounding areas.

Two related factors are also influential. On the one hand, the feeling of compassion and readiness to help results in a high degree of altruism; on the other, there is a considerable increase in criminality and manifestation of low moral principles. Mass evacuation and movement of refugees affects aspects of socioeconomic life, setting the stage for antisocial excesses. According to Babayeva [24], criminality among migrants in the USSR is three to four times that among permanent residents. In this atmosphere, as elsewhere, the activities of the staffs of health institutions are grounded in the principles of humanism and fidelity to the physicians' ethic, finding concrete expression in their participation in the choice of placement sites for the evacuated and refugees, and in observation of their adaptation to the local medical and geographical conditions and arrangements.

Public Health Care, Aid and Protection of the Population in Connection with Natural Disasters

Natural disasters are distinguished by their origin, their characteristics, and the extent of their effects. All these factors must be considered in drawing up measures of protection and aid for the stricken population, with the aim of reducing the consequences to a minimum. Modern scientific and technical achievements enable us to reach this aim. Considerable effort is needed, however, particularly with regard to material expenses for environmental sanitation. Priority must be given to the implementation of security measures. Of primary importance here, is overcoming the tendency to underestimate the effects of the disaster and their consequences, including those for public health.

Being relatively infrequent, disasters receive everyone's attention when they appear. In the course of time, however, watchfulness slackens. Much is forgotten until the appearance of another disaster causing death, mass traumatism, and greatly increased morbidity. In addition, in the process of unprecedented technical development, man has unwillingly created many harmful factors which have become further grounds for anthropogenic disasters [1].

Natural disasters of the present century have revealed the unreadiness of many countries to implement efficient protective and rescue measures (e.g., the Federal Republic of Germany, Italy, China, Morocco, Pakistan, Rumania, the USSR, Turkey, Yugoslavia, Chile, Japan). Only after a catastrophic earthquake on September 1, 1923, which took 100 000 lives did the Japanese erect towns with wide streets, seismically stable buildings, and an appropriate fire prevention system. In San Francisco in 1983 I observed to what extent the lessons of the earthquake on April 18–20, 1906 have been neglected; the earthquake caused widespread fires (Fig. 37 and 38). In the relatively narrow streets, wooden houses are built quite close to one another, among some stone constructions (Fig. 39). The approach to them is difficult, and cars filled with fuel are parked in rows on either side of the street. Considering the city's vulnerability to earthquakes, and its many hills and strong winds, this is an especially dangerous situation. It seems difficult to change the decades-old habit of arbitrary construction, which under normal conditions is justified to a certain extent by a more efficient use of local buildings materials, inexpensive buildings costs, and architectural traditions developed over generations.

The errors and defects are revealed only in an emergency situation. Measures are then undertaken, means are found, money is spent; what should have been done beforehand, in a normal and tranquil atmosphere, is done in haste and nervousness, amid mass injuries and heavy damages. This seems typical of countries throughout

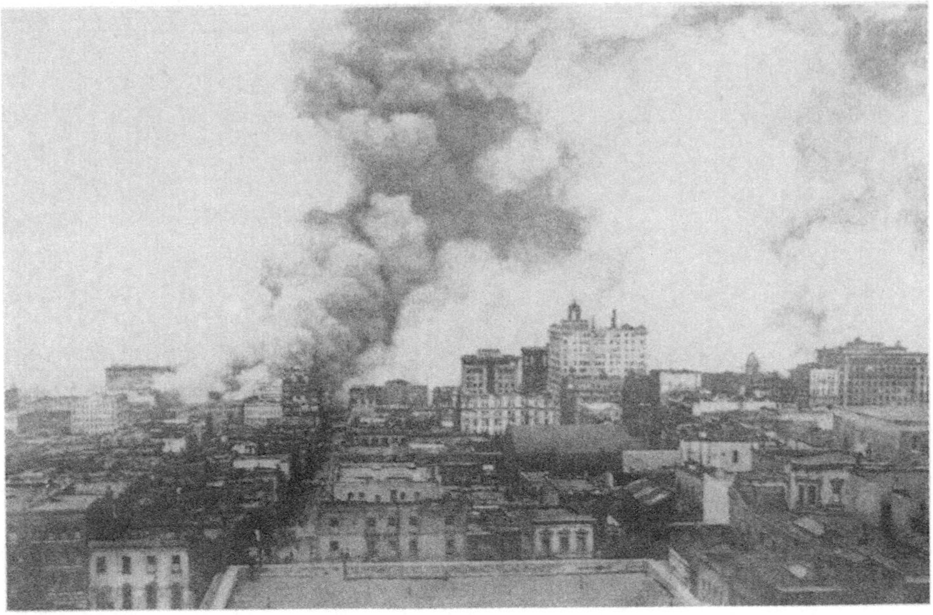

Fig. 37. Without water to fight the fires, San Francisco was doomed to burn [351]

the world, becoming a routine which must be accepted, though it ist generally acknowledged as unjustifiable.

The earthquake that destroyed Agadir (Morocco, 1960) showed that the town was ultimately unprepared for such a phenomenon [118]. From the medical campus I observed the destruction in Petropavlovsk-Kamchatsky (USSR) after the May 4, 1959 earthquake. This destruction was related to nonobservance of antiseismic requirements, and to construction errors [102]. The second earthquake (July 19, 1960) destroyed the settlement of Zhupanovo on Kronotski Bay, causing mass injuries (Fig. 40). Experts concluded that all stone buildings had been erected with a disregard for the very basic norms of construction [102]. The lessons of this disaster were not learned, however, and antiseismic measures were not implemented in other seismoactive regions of the USSR.

This especially concerns medical institutions and the systems of water supply and sewage disposal. Urazbayev et al. [254] state that the Tashkent earthquake of 1966 displayed the unreadiness of the local authorities to undertake antiseismic measures in building the municipal hospital no. 10, children's hospital no. 16, and the stomatology clinic. Almost 85% of the buildings of the Tashkent medical institutions, built without regard for the high seismic stability requirements, were damaged; 16% were put out of function entirely [62]. The same happened to residential buildings (Fig. 41).

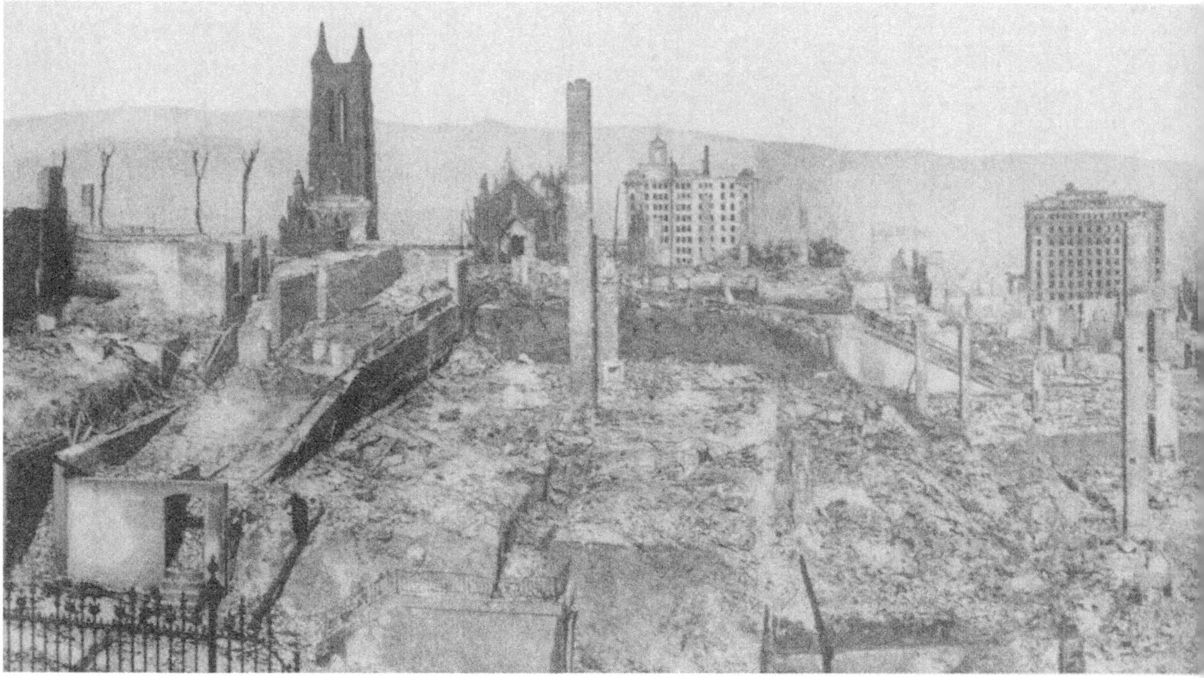

Fig. 38 *(bilon)*. San Francisco after the big fire [351]

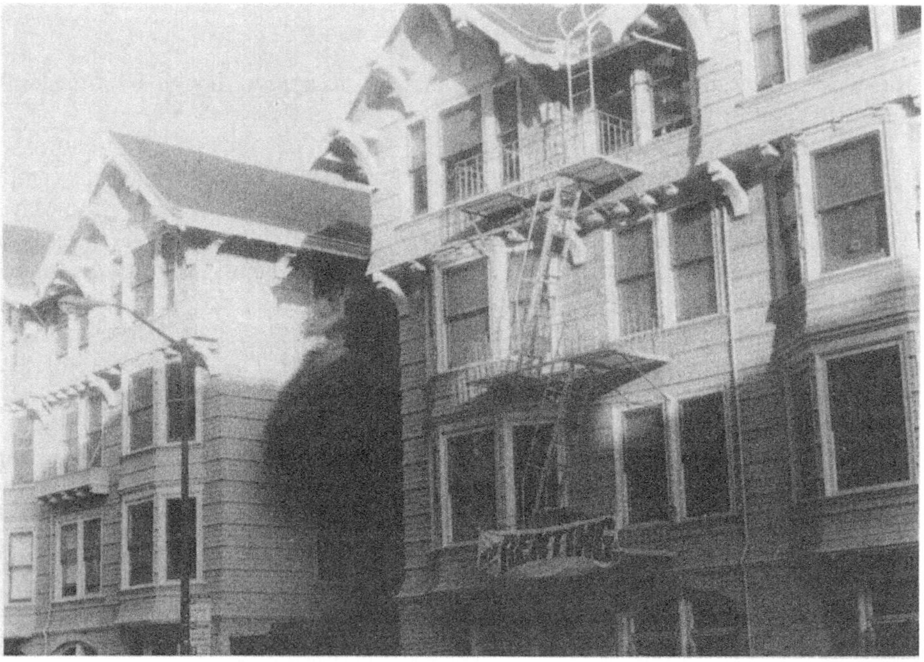

Fig. 39. Densely erected wooden houses in San Francisco (Author's photo)

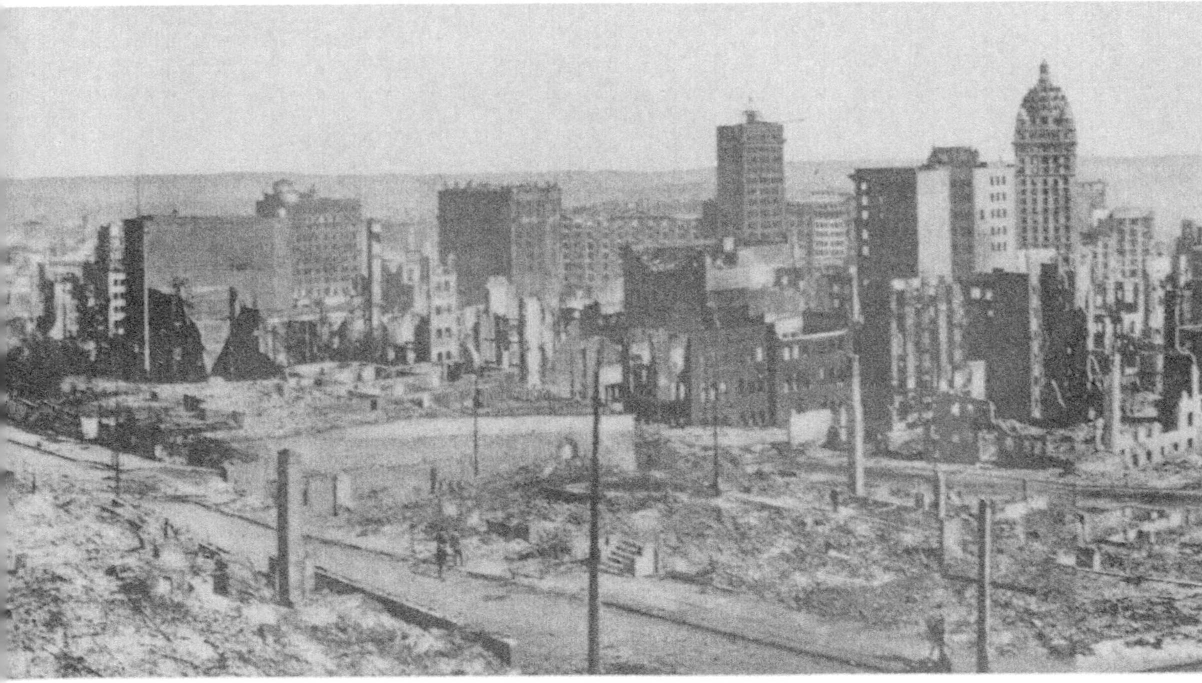

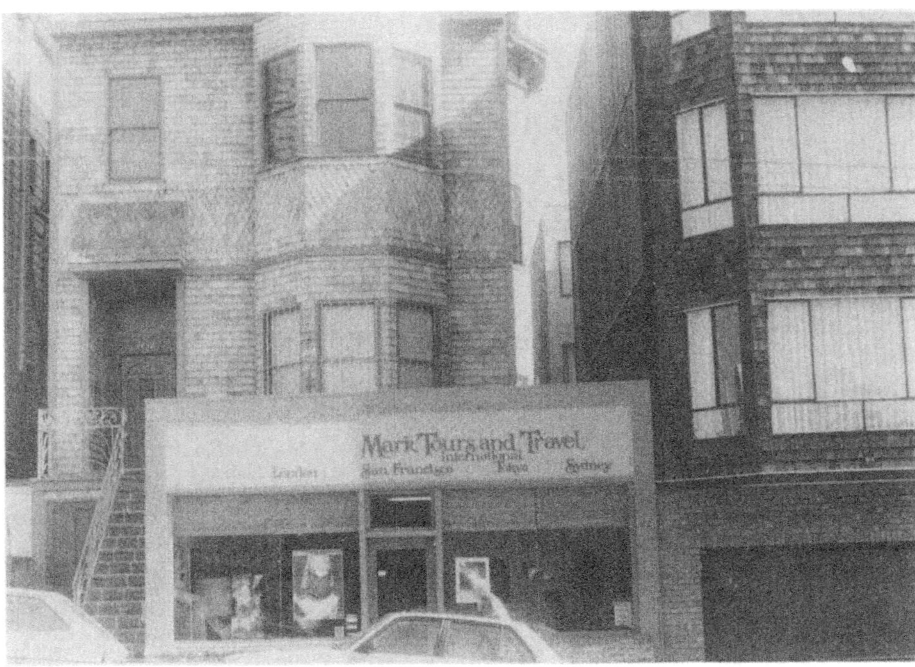

Fig. 39b.

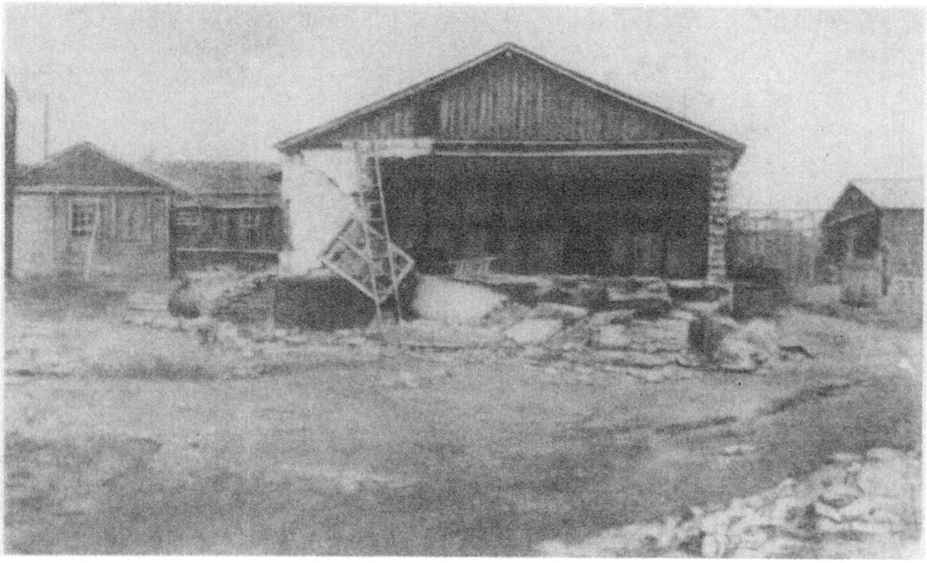

Fig. 40. Building in the settlement of Zhupanovo damaged by earthquake June 18, 1952 [102]

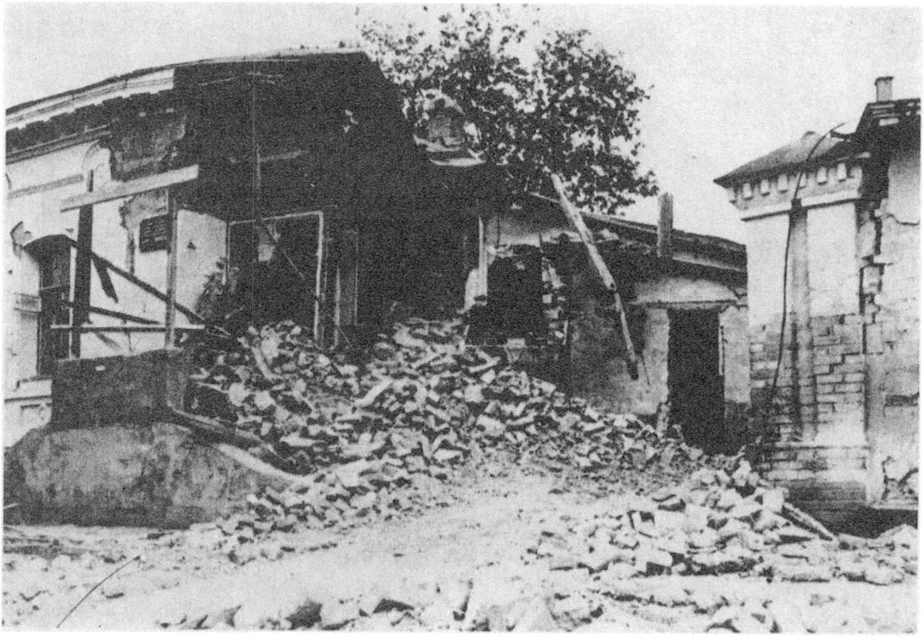

Fig. 41. Shakhrizabskaya Street, Tashkent, buildings destroyed on April 26, 1966 (G. Poun)

Table 39. Mortality among patients in Ashkhabad medical institutions during the earthquake of October 5, 1948

Institution	Mortality (%)
Children's Hospital for Infectious Diseases	100.0
Clinics of Turkmen Medical Institute	72.0
Psychiatric Hospital	64.0
Dermatologic and Venerologic Diseases (Regional) Dispensary (Children's Dept.)	42.6
Dermatologic and Venerologic Diseases Institute	28.0
Tuberculosis Dispensary (of the Republic)	25.0
Oncology Dispensary (of the Republic)	22.0
Trachoma Institute	20.0
Gastroenterologic Dispensary	20.0

Nazarov et al. [184] call attention to the low quality of construction and the violation of antiseismic norms, which resulted in serious damage to the polyclinic and the water supply and sewage systems in the settlement of Aronikh, and to the hotel in the settlement of Kadjaran, both of which were hit by the Zangezur (USSR) earthquake on June 9, 1968. And as a result of an earthquake on June 17, 1968, one-story buildings of both the children's and the adults' municipal hospitals in the town of Ismaill (Azerbaijan SSR) were badly damaged [16].

Lack of antiseismic provision when building hospitals in seismically dangerous zones is fraught with extremely grave consequences, as illustrated by the data in Table 39, compiled from reports on the Ashkhabad earthquake [347]. The highest number of deaths occured in the children's hospital, the clinics of the Turkmen Medical Institute, the psychiatric hospital, and the children's department of the regional dermatological-venerologic dispensary. Among the reasons which directly influenced (for the worse) the process of rescuing those being treated in the Ashkhabad hospitals are the following:

a) absence of rescue manpower and equipment,
b) the critical conditions of the patients, including postoperative,
c) the children's ages, determining their low levels of self-protection and self-aid capability,
d) the neuropsychological deviations of some patients, making them incapable of reacting appropriately to carry out rescue measures.

It is interesting to note that of the 189 who died outside San Francisco after the earthquake in 1906, 112 (59.2%) were patients at the Agnews Psychiatric Hospital near San Jose [215].

Thus, it is clear that medical institutions must be protected against the effects of possible natural disasters. In the United States, each medical institution has a plan for emergency situations, and drills for its practical implementation are exercised twice a year [113]. An important condition of the efficiency of such a plan is its coordination within the general system of health services, and the involvement of other institutions operative in the emergency situation caused by a natural disaster. It must be based on measures which are mostly of a preventive nature, and on actual circumstances.

In seismoactive zones the world over, disregard of antiseismic requirements in construction is frequent, and it is routinely observed in many countries vulnerable to natural disasters in the periods between two occurrences. Barannikov et al. [28] state that as a result of strong earthquakes in the municipal territory of Petropavlovsk-Kamchatsky in 1971 (reaching a magnitude of 8 on the Richter scale), the water supply and sewage systems were damaged in 21 places throughout the city. Investigation revealed that about half of the buildings were 50% uninhabitable.

Another country situated in a seismoactive zone, with quite another socio-economic structure, is Algeria. Nonetheless, with regard to the implementation of measures to protect against earthquakes the situation is similar to that in the USSR. In the El-Asama earthquake in 1954, 1600 people were killed. It might be supposed that once the consequences of the disaster had been eliminated and order restored, its lessons in terms of antiseismic measures to be implemented would have been apprehended. But this was not the case. In November 1980 an earthquake destroyed the town of El-Asam, and, according to press information, killed more than 20 000 people, and left 60 000 injured and 300 000 homeless.

Implementation of preventive measures is the responsibility of the authorities who set standards for stable construction, while the health services must assume the supervision and control functions. In addition, the health services are responsible for prophylactic measures against general and infectious diseases. Close study shows that here, too, the situation is far from satisfactory.

The flood which struck Staraya Russa in 1966 caused a drastic increase in infectious hepatitis (1.6 times higher than in the preceding year) and intestinal infections. Timely implementation of medical and prophylactic measures, including orderly supply of water to the town, undoubtedly could have diminished the public health consequences of this flood, at least with regard to the spread of the above mentioned diseases [34].

More than 10 years passed, and according to certain data, there had been hardly any improvement in the situation in the USSR. The Pskov region near Novgorod is also vulnerable to floods. We know that in such a situation the problems of contamination of water sources and provision of quality drinking water take on primary importance. For all that, according to Emelianova et al. [75], the high rate of intestinal infections was due to an unsatisfactory water supply system and continued pollution of open reservoirs – as registered in six administrative districts and two towns of the Pskov region. The typhoid morbidity was 2.9 per 1000 population (1974, 1975).

Some of the reasons for such a situation are:

1. The absence of a central authority responsible for supervision, organization, and implementation of preventive measures, protection, and aid to the population
2. Insufficiency or underestimation of information concerning the possibility of a natural disaster, its nature, effects, and the structure of injuries
3. A constant deficit of expert personnel and equipment for carrying out complicated projects to protect against natural disasters
4. Attitudinal drawbacks; an inclination to risk rather than meet the costs for preventive activities

Not least is the role played by a subjective factor: the lowering of moral principles. According to a 15 year plan elaborated by the municipal authorities of Los Angeles, 8000 buildings, determined to be unreliable in case of a magnitude-7 earthquake, were to have been reinforced or demolished. This would have reduced the estimated number of injured from 8000 to 1500 and the total number of people who in any way suffered from a disaster from 34 000 to 8000. Many home owners launched a protest against the program, which would have cost 750 million dollars. Residents and leaseholders were warned that if the plan were implemented they would be evicted or the rent would be drastically increased [186].

Instances of such neglect of security can be provided from other countries as well. Against a background of unprecedented destruction affecting the environment on a global scale, they reflect the crisis of man and culture, of placing greater interest in personal wealth than in humanistic values. Though apprehending the gravity of the price paid in lives and health, people prefer to assume responsibility for themselves rather than for society and mankind as a whole. Thus, the solution of medicoecological problems directly depends on the physical and spiritual improvement of man in the following areas: implementation of prophylactic measures of both an individual and a public nature, and interest in both the near future and the long-range perspective for mankind.

The modern world ist still far from realizing the above program. The English ecologist Nicolson is quite right in speaking of the "environmental revolution," which entails radical changes in our attitude towards the environment. It appears necessary to add here that a change of attitude is imperative in light of the potential dangers of natural disasters. In general, we assume that the problems lie in the social and economic disorders of many countries, and in the crisis in health services, which is closely connected with this disorder.

Seismologists, oceanologists, hydrologists, meteorologists, and other experts are all – within their professional frameworks – studying the reasons for and nature of earthquakes, tsunami, floods, mudflows and snow avalanches. They are developing methods of timely notification and efficient protective measures. Much has been achieved in scientific developments, but the medical aspects of the problem apparently remain underinvestigated.

Observation and supervision by the health services is unsatisfactory. For example, it took the May, 1960 earthquake in Chile to reveal the scandalously low quality of buildings in Valdivia, Puerto Monte, and Castro (including clinics, residences, and factories); they are made of cheap, low-quality concrete and low-quality steel and are erected on unreliable, shallow foundations [16]. In the town of Dijarbanir (southeast Turkey) a seven-story building inhabited by 150 people crashed during the night of January 2–3, 1983, killing 84 and injuring 44. The reason for the disaster was the low quality of the reinforced concrete. The building had been constructed by a contractor who was formerly employed as a worker at the municipal slaughterhouse. His employees were unqualified, and the entire construction was made without drawings and without any engineering supervision [348]. Thus, it is a broad system in which individuals or groups use their position, relying on a lack of controls, to expose people to danger for the sake of their own egotistical interests.

According to the theory of radical behaviorism, man as a creature is motivated by the sum of habits or habitual forms of behavior. This also concerns the problems of security. Today's physician is morally responsible for changing man's way of thinking and behaving up to the level at which individualism no longer conflicts with society's needs in the fight for a healthy environment. Manifestations of individualism may be rooted in various motives that may not be entirey clear. In this respect it is interesting to consider the data provided by Nozdrikov (in Toffler [273]) concerning road accidents in Moscow. They show that among drivers who had been working for more than 10 years, cases of traffic regulation violation increased. It is assumed that the reason for this is growing self-confidence. In addition, the number of people in this group killed in accidents as a result of drunken driving is three times greater than the average.

To prevent these phenomena from badly affecting public health security, there is a need for action by the appropriate state institutions, including legal force. With regard to environmental sanitation, the supervision and control functions of the health security organs must be directed toward:

1. Building of protective structures (dams, piers, breakwaters, afforestation); development of hydrotechnical projects to regulate the seasonal flow of water and the drainage of precipitation; observance of construction requirements, including antiseismic regulations; reconstruction and repair of old structures in seismoactive regions
2. Building of settlements on heights and in other safe places; planning of straight streets for fast evacuation (in tsunami-vulnerable regions)
3. Assignment of autonomous shelters with appropriate equipment for nontransportable patients from local medical institutions, as well as for other contingents of the population, including the homeless
4. Provision of an operative system for timely warning of approaching natural disasters, to be related with other protective and rescue services in accordance with plans made by municipal and state institutions
5. Provision of stable water supply and sewage systems for uninterrupted functioning, as well as standby emergency measures for disinfection of contamination sources
6. Preparation in advance of disaster, of rescue teams and specially assigned forces, including mobile medical aid groups and teams

The implementation of measures to combat natural disasters is a difficult and complex task. Primarily, it is connected with considerable material expenses, and resources are always limited. Their mobilization and use while the situation is normal involves overcoming the combination of inertia, carelessness, and skepticism. Only when the disaster strikes does the justification of the expenses become evident.

According to reports by the Tiraspol municipal authorities (Moldavia), total damages caused by the April 1959 flood came to 1 256 000 rubles. A works project connected with reinforcement of the riverbanks, which could have protected the town, had been estimated as costing 1 100 000 rubles, i.e., 12.5% less than the actual damages. Material losses due to the Guatemala earthquake of February 4, 1976 were estimated at one billion dollars [47]. In Italy, the Messina catastrophe has

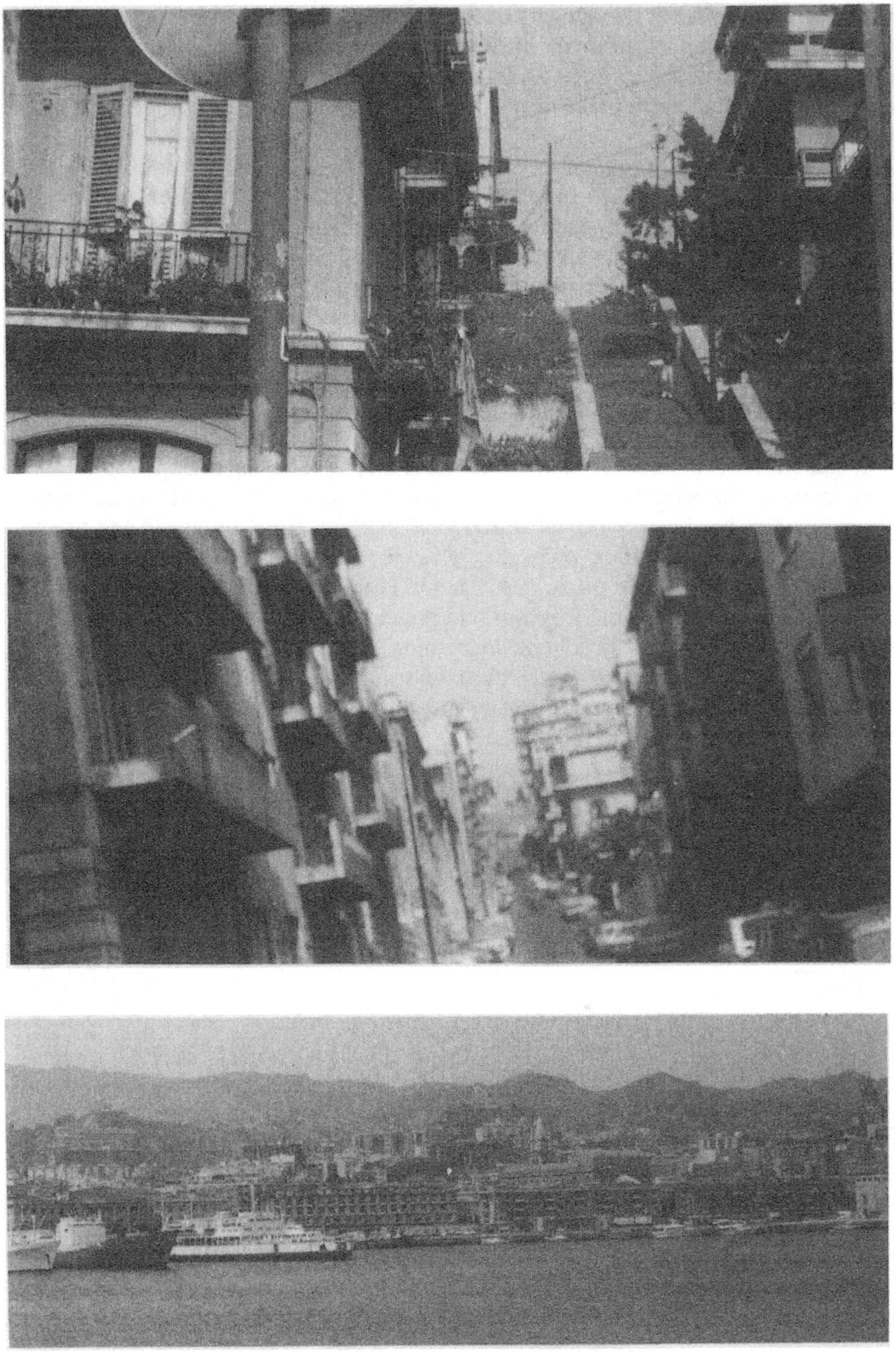

Fig. 42. Views of narrow streets with multistory houses and embankment, Messina, Italy, 1982 (Author's photo)

not been forgotten, but the dangers of the disaster, as illustrated by Fig. 42, showing narrow streets, the tsunami-vulnerable embankment of Messina, and multi-story buildings with balconies, were underestimated. It is not difficult to imagine the consequences of an earthquake or a tsunami, both of which are possible here, under these conditions.

Preventing these consequences is a part of environmental sanitation. There is a need to define the medicogeographical characteristics of any particular territory, but especially of extremely vulnerable zones. Taking into account the impact of natural factors on the life and health of people, definitions of districts of certain regions are necessary. Concerning earthquakes, special micro- and macro-regioning has been introduced in the USSR. The seismic regioning valid for 1967 is represented in Fig. 43, indicating the regions vulnerable to earthquakes of various magnitudes. There are also known tsunamogenic zones, as well as areas vulnerable to periodic flooding and mudflows. Thus, regional classification with regard to these natural disasters is also possible.

In general, it is possible to compile complex maps specifying regions vulnerable to earthquakes, tsunami, floods or other natural disasters. A certain recurrence of these disasters has been observed with regard to place, time, duration, and territory involved. There is nothing especially difficult about mapping potential natural disasters of anthropogenic origin. One should take into account

a) the possible extent of the territory and population involved,
b) the approximate prognostic data concerning the nature and structure of injuries,
c) the possible consequences for public health,
d) the probable time of its appearance (in light of known factors).

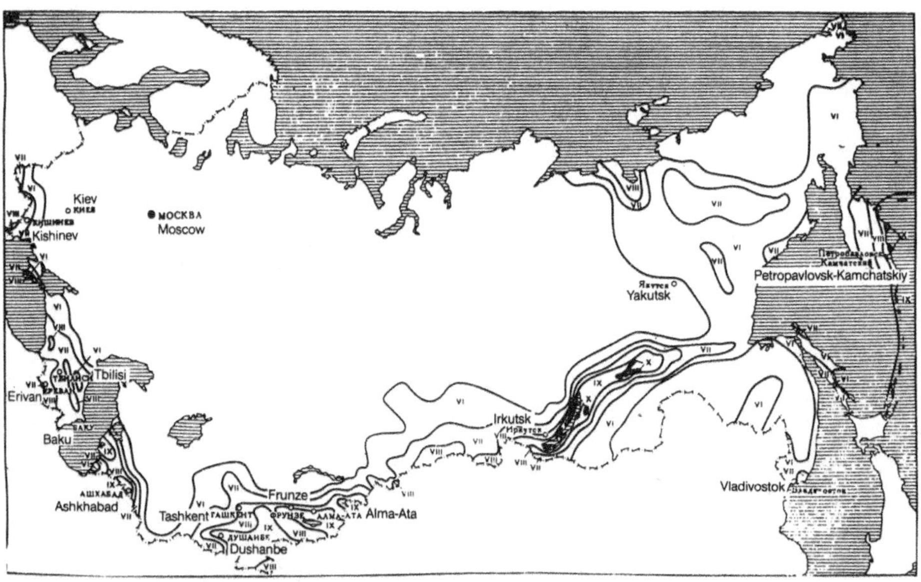

Fig. 43. Map of seismic regions of the USSR, 1967 (compiled in the Physics of Earth Institute, Academy of Sciences of the USSR). The numbers I to X denote regions of increasing frequency and intensity of earthquakes

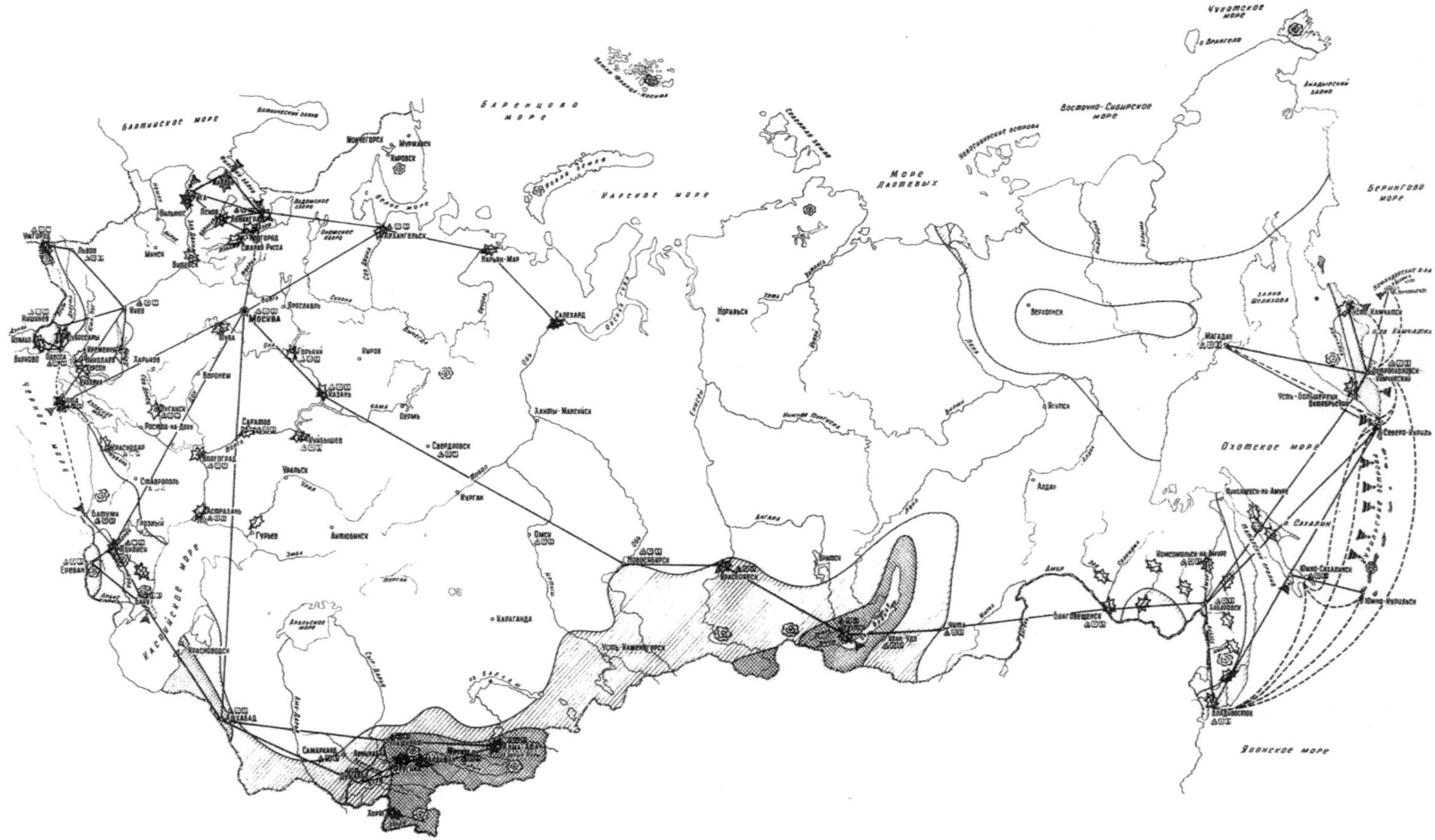

Fig. 44. Map and scheme for forecasting disasters with public health consequences, in the USSR

Determining the effects of a calamity and the structure of the consequences, particularly for public health, is dependent upon the peculiarities of recurrence. The information gathered from thorough investigation of natural disasters in various countries over many years must be the foundation of a regularly updated nosoprognostic medicogeographical map. Fig. 44 is an example of such a map applicable to the USSR. The map shows:

Character of natural disasters		Typical injuries, diseases	Projected time of occurrence
Earthquakes (score on Richter scale)	6–7 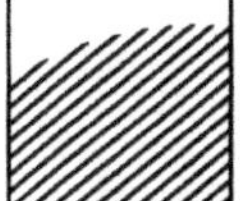	Traumatic injuries Aggravation of state of patients with chronic diseases, pregnant women, children, elderly people Increase in coronary attacks	Impossible to determine
	≥8 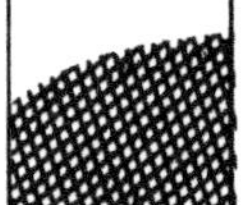	Traumatic injuries, burns, psychic disorders Infectious diseases (gastrointestinal, children's infections etc.) Aggravation of state of patients with chronic diseases, pregnant women, children, elderly people	
Floods	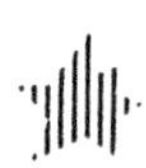	Diseases connected with cooling of environment (catarrhs of the respiratory tract, pneumonia, rheumatism etc.) Infectious diseases (dysentery, typhoid, paratyphoids, tularemia, children's infections) Slight injuries	Volkhov, Neva and other rivers of Novgorod, Leningrad, Pskov regions; Severnaya Dvina, Pechora and other rivers of Arkhangelsk region and Komi ASSR; Amu-Darya, Syr-Darya, and other rivers of Central Asia – spring-summer Dnieper, Dniester, other rivers of Ukrainian SSR and Moldavian SSR – spring Rivers of Far East, Danube – spring, summer, autumn
Tsunami	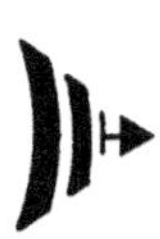	Drownings Traumatic injuries, psychic disorders Diseases connected with cooling of environment (catarrhs of the respiratory tract, pneumonia, rheumatism etc.) Infectious diseases (gastrointestinal, children's infections)	Impossible to determine
Mudflows		Traumatic injuries, drownings Diseases connected with cooling of environment Infectious diseases (gastrointestinal, children's infections).	Summer
Snow avalanches	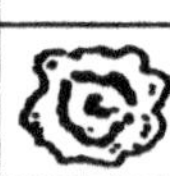	Traumatic injuries, frostbite Diseases connected with cooling of environment	Winter, winter-spring
	——— Aerial bridges	- - - - - Sea bridges	
Mobile medical aid groups		Mobile medical aid teams	Mobile antiepidemic teams

Principle Data on Medicogeographic Prognostication of Public Health Consequences of:

Earthquakes

Area vulnerable to earthquakes of magnitude 6–10 – 28.6% of USSR

For a 60–80-year period the strongest earthquakes took place in the following seismic regions: Precarpathian region, 4; Crimea, 4; Caucasus, 9; Kopet-Dag, 4; other regions of Central Asia, 14; Baikal region, 3; Far East, 7; total, 45

Traumatic injuries by severity (as percentage of total traumatic injuries): slight traumas, 62–94%; medium to severe traumas, 6–10%; crush syndrome, 3.5–79% of those with fractures of tubular bones; killed, 0.45–28.6%; killed, died of injuries sustained during earthquake, up to 14% of total population of region

Medical aid needed (% of cases): surgery, 65; general medicine, 12; opthalmology, 11; pediatrics, 7; obstetrics-gynecology, 5

Evacuated: with traumatic injuries, 95%; in connection with diseases, 5%; severely injured among evacuated: 5% of total population

Classification of injured needing hospital treatment (%): injuries of soft tissues with extensive hemorrhaging, 32; fractures of upper and lower extremities, 17–20; head traumas, 15–38; spine traumas, 3–5; pelvis and pelvic bone injuries, 4; injuries of organs of abdominal cavity, 0.2; others, 27

Increase in mortality of hospitalized patients in earthquake zone (max. % increase): obstetrics-gynecology, 200; stillbirths, 50; general children's diseases, 50; general medicine, 40; infectious diseases, 40; surgery, 30; psychiatry, 1700

Tsunami

General characteristic: mass injuries in a short period of time

Ratio of injured to killed: 1:0.22 to 1:2.9

Killed: by drowning, 11%; washed into sea, 50–60%

Increased delivery of patients to hospitals (%): opthalmology, 128; gynecology, 124; otolaryngology, 123; general medicine, 119; infectious disease (children, 105, adults, 117); surgery, 104

Increase in admission of patients to hospitals (max. % increase): pneumonia, 60; traumas, 50; gastrointestinal diseases, 50; urinary system diseases, 50

Increase in mortality (%): children's infectious diseases, 159; surgery, 114; gynecological diseases, 112

Increase in mortality of patients treated at home: traumas, up to 240%; pneumonia, up to 200%

Floods

General characteristics: mass injuries in a short period of time; large numbers left homeless; considerable territory involved

Increase in diseases directly as a result of the flood: traumas, 2–10 times; pneumonia, 4 times; rheumatism, 3 times; catarrhs of respiratory tract, tonsillitis (in children can increase up to 40%, including pneumonia cases; cases of measles and scarlet fever, 10.4%), 1.5 times; gynecologic diseases, 1.5 times as much

Increase in infectious diseases: whooping cough, 9 times; scarlet fever, 4 times; typhoid, 4 times; measles, 4 times; epidemic parotitis, double

1. Seismoactive zones with potentially strong earthquakes (magnitude 6–7 to 9–10)
2. Regions with possible tsunami of seismic and meteorological origin of groups 3, 4, and 5 (according to Imamura's classification)
3. Territories with possible typhoons, floods, mudflows, and snow acalanches (of medium and considerable degrees of danger)
4. Approximate timing of the appearance of natural disasters (tsunami, floods, mudflows, snow avalanches)
5. The structure and composition of injuries, diseases (somatic and infectious), caused by the effects of the disaster and the unfavorable environmental conditions
6. Regions assigned for placement of the evacuated population, the injured, and the homeless in need of safe shelters
7. Medical forces involved (it is desirable to indicate the place and time of their formation, dispatch, activities, the composition of staff and equipment)
8. Routes and means of delivering medical personnel and equipment to the disaster site, and for evacuation of the injured and ill to medical institutions

The characteristics of earthquakes are indicated in the table and legend accompanying Fig. 44 by:
1. The number of strong earthquakes which have taken place in the past 60–80 years in the seismic zones of the USSR
2. The approximate composition of traumatic injuries according to the degree of severity and the type of medical aid needed
3. The group of injured needing evacuation
4. The structure of injuries and need for hospitalization
5. The possible increase in hospital mortality

The characteristics of tsunami are indicated by:
1. The ratio of killed to injured
2. The possible proportion of those drowned and swept out to sea
3. The dynamics of delivery of patients to hospitals in connection with various diseases
4. Increased mortality

The characteristics of floods are indicated by:
1. The extent and proportion of various types of injuries
2. Increase in morbidity and traumatism caused by the flood and overcooling
3. Increase in infectious mobidity

In connection with hydrotechnical construction, we encounter diseases such as malaria, tularemia, ixodiasis, and rickettsiosis asiatica. Engineering projects meant to protect settlements from floods sometimes become responsible for the formation of shoals and water stagnation in pools, which to a certain extent promotes the appearance of these diseases. Such projects must therefore be supervised by the health authorities, and mapping of these regions is of organizational importance.

The above serves as an orientation for compilation of nosoprognostic medicogeographical maps of natural disasters. They are needed for:

a) environmental sanitation,
b) timely implementation of projects to prevent the effects of natural disasters, and to protect against them,
c) planning of medical aid to the injured and estimation of manpower and means needed, and limitation of the public health consequences of natural disasters.

In terms of the territory involved, the nosoprognostic maps may be:
1. Small-scale (1 : 1 000 000), covering the entire country
2. Medium-scale (1 : 500 000, 1 : 200 000), covering large administrative regions
3. Large-scale (1 : 50 000, 1 : 25 000), covering individual districts in great detail

Since one of the characteristic features of natural disasters is their sudden appearance, the importance of detail in prognostication and mapping of their public health consequences cannot be overestimated. This concerns above all the amount of personnel and medical equipment needed. From my own experience and from the materials I have studied, I am led to conclude that medical forces and means arrive at the site of a disaster with considerable delay. Data on the Ashkhabad earthquake illustrate this point [349] (Fig. 45 [32]). The majority of the medical personnel arrived in Ashkhabad on the second day after the earthquake; a considerable contingent did not arrive until the third day. The reason for this were
a) insufficient preparation and provision of equipment for the various forces and for their dispatch, and
b) errors in transmission of quick, relatively comprehensive, and reliable information on the disaster because of malfunctions in the communication system, the death, illnes, or resignation of people responsible for communication, or specific considerations of certain authorities.

The writer Lazar Karelin [129] vividly depicts how people in the USSR were informed of the Ashkhabad quake: "He did not believe this horrible news. Still he switched on the loudspeaker, waiting for the newscast. The news items followed one another, but no word was pronounced with regard to the Ashkhabad earthquake.

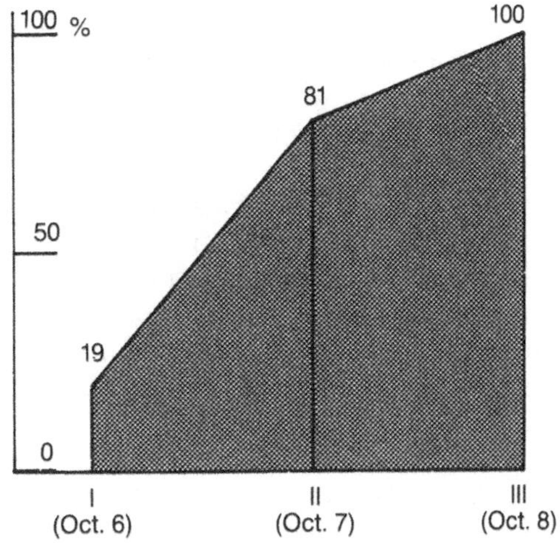

Fig. 45. Arrival of medical personnel in Ashkhabad (1948) for management of the public health consequences of earthquake

How could it be? Anyway, something must have happened there. He knew nothing about earthquakes, but what he did know was the sad science of hushing-up, into which many events were enveloped as if they never happened. And people studied the art of guessing, which replaced the notion of 'perceiving news'; they studied how to live with rumors, instead of news."

Natural disasters almost always come suddenly, and the atmosphere in the stricken zone becomes depressing [34]; the feeling of fear sometimes leads to madness. For the medical personnel of Tashkent the most difficult problem was protecting the population from the neuropsychical reactions and their various complications [155].

After the eartquake of January 15, 1968 in Sicily, as reported by the press, 600 000 people of Palermo spent two nights outside, in panic, chaos, and mass hysteria. The residents who had been left homeless badly needed bread, water, shelter, and medical treatment. All these facts must be considered when the public health institutions begin to plan for coping with natural disasters.

On the basis of investigations and personal experience I am convinced that, in a wider sense, medical personnel are not sufficiently acquainted with the problem, in spite of the practical interest shown by medical institutions. This is especially relevant for those zones known to be vulnerable to natural disasters. To change this situation, in addition to training experts to deal with the consequences of accidents and disasters, there is a need to organize special training and drills for general medical personnel within the framework of the public health security services. This training should cover:

1. The organization of medical aid to the injured, taking into account the mass nature of the injuries and the limitations of time, forces and means; care of patients with chronic diseases and pregnant women with the use of mobile medical aid teams and functional subdivisions at separate medical posts, in cooperation with the health authorities of adjacent towns [31]
2. The detection of patients having or suspected of having infectious diseases, to isolate or hospitalize them and then implement antiepidemic measures
3. The use of standardized methods of treatment, reanimation, and surgical interference according to vital indications
4. The cooperation between different teams under public health service authorities, military health services, medical subdivisions of the civil defense authorities, and others, to provide coherence to the activities with regard to the specific geographical conditions

The experiences of China and Indonesia justify the training of people for primary medicosanitary services. In addition, the population itself must be trained in techniques of self-aid and mutual aid.

Upon implementation of protection measures and rescue activities, different groups of the population (as planned beforehand) carry out different work and are responsible for different functions according to their position, type, and character of activities, special knowledge and experience, and physical capabilities. In this respect, special training, in addition to the general preparation given to the whole population (as, for example, techniques of self-aid and mutual aid for various injuries) must envisage both theoretical and practical studies of the problems

Table 40. The complex of measures related to natural disasters, as implemented by health authorities

Measures implemented	Natural disasters		
	Earthquakes	Tsunami	Floods
Public health and safety			
Participation of public health physicians in planning towns and settlements, taking into account:			
Possible injurious effects of natural disasters	+	+	+
Fire protection	+		
Optimal evacuation of population in case of emergency	+	+	+
Determination of places for launching dispensation of medical aid	+	+	+
Possible modification of relief in connection with planning various constructions	+	+	
Supervision of construction activities with attention to increased seismic stability in response to manipulation of local environment	+		
Supervision of construction of dams and security measures for settlements on big rivers		+	+
Supervision of			
Building of protective constructions, protective afforestation		+	+
Works connected with bank reinforcement			+
Supervision of construction, maintenance, and exploitation of water supply, sewage systems, and natural wells	+	+	+
Supervision of placement and exploitation of industrial enterprises and hydroelectric constructions	+	+	+
Supervision of establishment of water reservoirs, electricity and heating supply reserves	+	+	+
Supervision of building, and maintenance of temporary shelters, places for evacuated	+	+	+
Antiepidemic			
Epidemiologic assessment of the situation	+	+	+
Struggle against intestinal infections			
Implementation of measures related to general state of public health and specific prophylaxis	+	+	+
Implementation of measures related to manifestation of intestinal infectious diseases	+	+	+
Struggle against children's infectious diseases (diphtheria, chickenpox, measles, whooping cough, mumps, scarlet fever):			
General measures	+	+	+
Measures for preventing spread of children's infectious diseases	+	+	+
Detection and elimination of sources of tularemia			
General sanitary measures		+	+
Vaccination of total population where indicated		+	+
Detection and elimination of sources of leishmaniasis	+		
Detection and elimination of sources of leptospirosis			
General sanitary measures	+	+	+
Vaccination where indicated		+	+

Table 40. (continued)

Measures implemented	Natural disasters Earthquakes	Tsunami	Floods
Treatment, prophylaxis			
Psychotherapy	+	+	+
Dispensary observation of cardiovascular patients	+	+	+
Treatment of patients with myocardial infarction, cardiopulmonary insufficiency, and respiration and nutrition problems	+	+	+
Dispensary observation of patients with: rheumatism, diabetes mellitus, gastric and duodenal ulcers, cholecystitis, gynecological problems, psychological problems, etc.	+	+	+
Organizational			
Preparation of teams for activities in the zone of the natural disaster	+	+	+
Preparation of medical institutions for receiving large numbers of injured, with the following cases prevailing:			
Injured women and children	+	+	+
Those rescued from water (with corporal overcooling)		+	+
Compound problems	+	+	+
Preparation of medical institutions for receiving large numbers of patients with traumatic injuries, with the following cases prevailing:			
Fractures of extremities	+	+	+
Skull traumas; traumas of spine, pelvis, and thorax	+		
Extended injuries of soft tissue, including effects of prolonged squashing	+		
Burns	+		
Preparation of medical institutions with respect to:			
Evacuation of patients	+	+	+
Organization of autonomous shelters for nontransportable patients		+	+
Public health provisions for evacuated population	+	+	+
Elaboration of medical aid plan and elimination of public health consequences of the natural disaster	+	+	+
Special training of medical personnel in:			
Launching formations assigned for implementation of activities in the disaster zone	+	+	+
Rendering medical aid at different stages of evacuation	+	+	+
Antiepidemic provisions	+	+	+
Public health and safety instructions to population with attention to:			
First aid (within self-aid and mutual aid)	+	+	+
Appropriate behavior under conditions of natural disaster	+	+	+
Life saving instruction in the event of being washed out to sea		+	
Scientific-research activities in relation to natural disasters	+	+	+
Compilation of nosoprognostic maps of territories vulnerable to natural disasters	+	+	+
Development of liaison between military medical services, civil health authorities, and voluntary organizations (Red Cross and Red Crescent organizations and others)	+	+	+

relating to the specific functional responsibilites of particular services, including those of the civilian national guard (rescue, evacuation, fire fighting, medical).

In areas vulnerable to tsunami, floods, and mudflows there is a need to train rescue teams in the various techniques for the rescue of people from drowning and in providing them with first aid. The medical personnel included in these teams should be proficient in reanimation techniques.

Special medical training does not have to take on the character of a campaign. It should constitute an integral part of systematically implemented activities headed by authorities responsible for health security services in case of natural disasters. The program for training experts in providing protection and aid must include such areas as probability theory, decision-making, and principles of management. A multi-branch institute for environmental studies should be established [87]. Table 40 is a summary of the content and character of the activities specified above.

Purposefully directed activities of the health authorities in connection with natural disasters can mean

a) prevention and protection,
b) the possiblity to counter the tragedy of a disaster with organized preparedness of manpower and means to assist the injured and to eliminate the consequences for public health, and
c) keeping the number of injured to a minimum and reduction of the gravity of the consequences.

This is the real aim of the health authorities with respect to natural disasters.

Conclusion

Natural disasters are a complex problem for the entire world. Most of all this concerns countries with seismically active and tsunamogenic zones, which increase the potential for floods, mudflows, snow avalanches, and other damaging phenomena of nature.

Their appearance is determined by the impact of both nature and man's activities, and cannot be accounted for by the regular laws of nature. The anthropogenic reconstruction of the natural environment directly effects

a) geographical factors, especially those of an extreme nature,
b) population distribution and the traditional character, conditions, and rhythm of everyday life,
c) industrial and agricultural development and the use of energy and other natural resources,
d) the health of the entire population.

Natural disasters interfere suddenly in all spheres of life, bringing about drastic changes in routine for a certain period of time. They also cause considerable long-term damage and have public health and other unexpected consequences. To a great extent, their scope and character are determined by the socioeconomic disorder of a country, which makes the situation even more complicated and acute. A natural disaster lays bare the latent malfunctions of the public and state organizations and institutions. It also reveals the impulse of altruism, people's feelings of compassion and their readiness to help victims. Medical deontology takes on a special significance.

The loss of a proper perspective in the absence of preparedness lays the ground for a critical situation. The factor of suddenness plays a special role. The beginning of a disaster is of special importance as far as organization of rescue activities and emergency measures are concerned. Efficient handling of the problems that arise and prevention of complications during this period are possible only if manpower and materials are available immediately and have been prepared in advance.

Such measures depend on data documenting the territories which are vulnerable, the conditions for the appearance of a natural disaster, knowledge of its first signs, its character, and the structure of the injuries it causes. Valuable prognostic material is provided by historical studies of natural disasters and how they were handled, and by analysis of the errors comitted. These errors recur from one calamity to the next, the reason being the persistent lack of material and means, and the manifest passiveness and carelessness of people up to the very moment that the emergency occurs. People tend to underestimate the importance of preventive measures and the indispensability of being constantly prepared.

In essence, the problem is one of providing security to the population of a country in the widest sense. Actions aimed at securing the future at the state level must overcome the personal egoistic interests that currently prevail. It is necessary for the people to learn to live with certain self-restrictions, as the problem is not only one of nature, but also of man's activities. It is inadmissable that chaos develops alongside rationalism. The tendency to the maximal use of energy and other natural resources, to scientific achievements in the fields of genetics and space research, ignores the background of unsolved social problems and the considerable lag in environmental sanitation. It is not by chance that the American futurologist Alvin Toffler [273] writes about the danger of electron smog, informational pollution, cosmic war, genetic filtration, climatic intervention, and ecological war having the potential to artificially cause earthquakes, tsunami, and floods.

In acting to change this situation, one must consider the geographical, historical, and socioeconomic peculiarities of a country and the considerable impact of the people's activities, mode of life, and psychological and moral-ethical principles.

Where natural disasters are concerned, different countries are differently involved in similar problems, and are at different levels in solving them. In several countries (and their number is constantly growing) hunger and malnutrition have become the routine accompaniment to swift population growth. In others, the growth of the transportation network and the increase in traffic are accompanied by a growing number of road accidents and their ensuing injuries. Taking on a mass character, these have become a nationwide disaster of anthropogenic origin. The preventive measures undertaken do not constitute a comprehensive answer to the principal causes of road accidents, and remain insufficient, as is the case with other types of natural disasters.

This study has provided the characteristics and structural peculiarities of earthquakes, tsunami, floods, mudflows, snow avalanches, hunger, and road traffic accidents. Provision of medical aid within the limitations encountered is of utmost importance to preserve lives and prevent serious sanitary consequences.

During the initial period of a disaster it is impossible to provide the aid of a physician for all those in need of it, due to the shortage of medical manpower and means. Under such conditions, first aid to oneself and one's fellow victims takes on special significance. Thus, the main point is that of medical self-help, which is widely useful in everyday life as well. Many people learn and carry out in practice basic medical procedures quite successfully (measuring arterial pressure, treating minor injuries, etc.). First aid is followed by aid from paramedics, and then from specialists.

On the basis of my own experience, I propose the organization of the following teams to be dispatched to a disaster area:

a) mobile medical aid groups,
b) mobile medical aid teams, capable of providing qualified medical and surgical aid according to vital indications,
c) mobile antiepidemic teams.

The present study details the extent and character of medical aid provided to the injured at different stages of a disaster, as well as the formation of medical aid groups and the work they do with the appropriate equipment, prepared and assigned especially for this purpose by medical and other institutions under the direction of the governmental health authorities.

Provision of medical aid is interconnected with the evacuation of the injured and the ill, and with the care of the evacuated population. On the basis of a special classifcation of the population, I have here recommended a scheme for medical provision, oriented with regard to which medical forces and means should be used at each stage of the evacuation, and to the character and extent of medical measures necessary, depending on the amount of time available.

This work has also dealt with the activities of the health authorities, including preventive sanitary-hygienic, sanitary antiepidemic, treatment-prophylactic, and organizational measures. The effectiveness of such measures depends on prognostic data, illustrated by the mapped prognostic schemes of public health consequences which I have elaborated for natural disasters within the territory of the USSR.

Similar nosoprognostic maps can provide health security institutions with a basic for countermeasures to the predicted disasters. Further action on a nationwide level, based on modern scientific and technical achievements, will make it possible to minimize the effects of natural disasters, and to reduce the gravity of their consequences, including those for public health.

References

1. Abbou (1972) Consequences de pollutione et des nuisances sur la sante publique. Rev Secur 8 (83):38–46
2. Abdianis (1948) Earthquake in Iran. Nature 162 (4121):647–648
3. Abdullayev AA, Karpova VL (1970) Detailed course of myocardial infarction with reference to a clinical sample. In: Proceedings of 44th Scientific Conference of Researchers of the Professional Advance Institute for Physicians, Tashkent, pp 21–22 (in Russian)
4. Alekseyev AA (1966) Details of clinical treatment of typhoid and evaluation of immunological research methods – a regional perspective. Transactions of the 9th Republican Congress of Medical Personnel of the Kirghiz SSR, Frunze, pp 469–474 (in Russian)
5. Alekseyev GK (1982) Innovations in intensive therapy and reanimation in medical practice (in Russian). Clin Med 8:116–119
6. Alimov KA, Vaserfirer NN (1967) Neurophysical reactions of healthy people and those with somatic diseases to the Tashkent earthquake. Thesis of report delivered at scientific conference on research related to the Tashkent quake of April 26, 1966, and its recurrent tremors, Tashkent, pp 42–43 (in Russian)
7. Alland A (1968) War and disease, an anthropological perspektive. Bull Atomic Scientists 24 (6):28–31
8. Ambraseys NN (1966) Seismic environment. The Skopje earthquake of July 1963. Rev Union Int Secours 5:62–82
9. Angelbert M, Reiss R (1980) Injuries of thorax and abdomen. Harefuah 98 (9):424–425
10. Antrushin IS (1961) The struggle against floods (in Russian). Priroda 11:103–104
11. Ariel MB, Kleonsky EE (1951) Tuberculosis and disturbances in nutrition. Experience of Soviet medicine in the great patriotic war (1941–1945). vol 25, pp 206–237. Medgiz, Moscow (in Russian)
12. Aripov UA (1969) Experience in organization of medical aid to the population of Tashkent during the period of elimination of the 1966 earthquake consequences (in Russian). Med Zh Uzb 7:83–85
13. Armand D (1970) The anxiety is justified, the hopes are real (in Russian). Literaturnaya Gazeta, Feb. 25, No 9
14. Armelagos G, Katz P (1977) Technology, health, and disease in America. Ecologist 7 (7):304–317
15. Arturo Romero B, Cobar R, Western KA, Lopez SM (1978) Some Epidemiological features of disasters in Guatemala. Disasters 2 (1):39–46
16. Asamirzayev RA, Djafarov RD, Giul EK, Zolotovitskaya TA (1972) The Ismailinsk earthquakes of February 5 and 9 and June 17, 1968. In: Earthquakes in the USSR, Nauka, Moscow, pp 21–34 (in Russian)
17. Assar M (1971) Guide to sanitation in natural disasters. World Health Organization, Geneva
18. Atakhanov EI, Turakulov YK (1958) Modern problems of regional pathology in Uzbekistan (in Russian). Clin Med 36 (6):3–8
19. Atakhanov EI (1963) Enterocolitis in a hot climate, and changes of certain metabolic indices (in Russian). Vestnik AMN SSSR 10:42–48
20. Atwater M (1968) The avalanche hunters. Philadelphia

21. Avtsyn AP (1966) Problems of geographical pathology in extreme zones (in Russian). Vestnik AMN SSSR 11:53–58
22. Avtsyn AP (1972) Introduction to geographical pathology. Meditzina, Moscow (in Russian)
23. Avo HH (1974) Auf dem Weg zur Erdbeben-Prognose. Kunst und Literatur, Stuttgart, 11:1159–1163
24. Babayev MM (1975) Demography and law (in Russian). Vopr Filos I:61–63
25. Bakhadyrov AB, Koroliov GP (1974) Distribution and mortality of myocardial infarction among the population of several Tashkent districts (in Russian). Med Zh Uzb 1:51–55
26. Bagramov L (1977) Food provision and policy (in Russian). Mezhdunar Zhizn 5:51–60
27. Bazhenow N (1914) On the significance of natural disasters in the etiology of some neuroses and psychoses (in Russian). SS Kocsakov. J Neuropatol Psikhiatr 1–2:1–14
28. Barannikov LB, Borisova NS, Yershov IA, Konstantinova TG, Medvedev SV, Fedotov SA, Fedianova SN, Shteinberg VV, Shumilin LS (1975) Macroscopic investigation of the consequences of the November 24–25, 1971 earthquake on the territory of the city of Petropavlovsk-Kamchatskij. In: Strong Kamchatka earthquakes, Vladivostok, pp 15–62 (in Russian)
29. Barlow EW (1955) Krakatoa 1883. Mar Obs 25 (170):221–227
30. Beinin LA (1954) Experience of the organization of medical examination of railway military personnel (in Russian). Voyenno-Med Zh 7:56
31. Beinin LA (1968) On the injuring effect of tsunami and principles of organization of medical aid to the injured (in Russian). Sov Med 4:137–140
32. Beinin L (1970) Natural calamities as a problem of geographical pathology, medical geography and public health organization (in Russian). Dissertation, Moscow
33. Beinin L (1978) Sanitary consequences of inundations, and medical care. First International Conference on Mass Casualty Management, September 17–20, 1978, Safed, Israel, p 32
34. Beinin L (1979) Sanitary consequences of inundations. Disasters 3 (2):213–216
35. Beinin L (1981) An examination of health data following two major earthquakes in Russia. Disasters 5 (2):142–146
36. Beinin S (1982) Road accidents – a problem of public health in Israel. Dissertation, Tel Aviv
37. Belousov V, Ibi G, Karus E, Linekhan D, Takeyama K (1962) Report of the UNESCO Seismological Mission to Southeast Asia, Australia, and the islands of the Pacific Ocean (in Russian). Moscow
38. Bevza GG, Bevza KP, Vinovatov YI, Diskalenko AP, Strokataya VI, Tzank VD (1971) Hydrological and hygienic characteristics of the Dniester River within the borders of Moldavia. In: Problems of meteorological investigations. Hydrometeoizdat, Moscow, vol 120, p 156 (in Russian)
39. Bigelow HB, Edmondson WT (1947) Wind waves, sea breakers, and surf. Washington
40. Boiko VM (1967) The problem of organization of sanitary antiepidemic measures during the period of elimination of the earthquake consequences in Tashkent (in Russian). In: Proceedings of the 4th scientific congress on urgent problems of infectious pathology, Tashkent, pp 63–65
41. Boldanov EV (1969) International symposium of floods and their prediction. Hydrometeoizdat, Leningrad p 625
42. Boltenstern T (1962) Die Situation im Hamburger Katastrophengebiet und die Flutkatastrophe vom 17. 2. 1962 aus der Sicht des Tiefbauingenieurs. Mun Med Wochenschr 42:1974–1978
43. Bombard A (1958) Overboard of his own free will, chap 8. Inostr Literatura, Moscow, p 8 (in Russian)
44. Borgstrom G (1971) Too many. An ecological overview of earth's limitations. Collier-Macmillan, New York, p XV
45. Brusilovsky LY, Bruchansky NP, Segalov TE (1928) The Crimean earthquake and neuropsychic traumas (in Russian). Narkomzdrav, RFSSR
46. Buldrini A, Lyppi A, Bucci G (1967) La morbosità per alcune malattine infettive nella provincia di Rovigo durante il decennio 1956–1965. Tech Sanit 5 (3):333–350
47. Bune VI (1977) Seismic regioning and estimation of seismic risk (in Russian). Phizika Zemli 7:109–112

48. Burdenov AS (1977) Mountainous countries and natural sources of plague. In: Ecological methods of study and organization of mammals' protection in mountainous areas. Sverdlovsk, pp 28–29 (in Russian)
49. Chaika EM (1951) Pathological anatomy of alimentary dystrophy. Experience of Soviet medicine in the great patriotic war (1941–1945), vol 28. Medgiz, Moscow (in Russian) pp 56–88
50. Casberg MA, Washington MD (1954) Medical organization in national catastrophes. JAMA 154 (6):501–506
51. de Castro J (1954) Geography of hunger. Moscow (in Russian)
52. Cech J, Smolensky M, Lane R, Halevy B, Samueloff S (1977) Meteorologic factors and temporal variations of cardiac mortality in an urban setting in a desert climatic zone. Isr J Med Sci 13 (5):451–459
53. Chornaya GF (1970) The course of hypertensive crises under the stress caused by an earthquake. Proceedings of the scientific conference dedicated to the 50th anniversary of the Tashkent State Medical Institute, Tashkent, pp 27–30 (in Russian)
54. Cherkheulidze II (1967) Protecting and regulating constructions of prefabricated ferro-concrete near mountain rivers. Hydrometeoizdat, Leningrad (in Russian)
55. Chodjayev SK (1971) Urgent problems of antiepidemic services during the period of liquidation of the earthquake's sanitary consequences in Tashkent. In: The Tashkent earthquake of April 26, 1966. Tashkent, pp 626–628 (in Russian)
56. Dolgatov I (1970) Today's problems (in Russian). Daghestanskaya Pravda, July 1, No 152
57. Davison C (1931) The Japanese earthquake of 1923. London
58. Deussen I (1962) Über Entstehung und Bekämpfung der Panik, part 1. Wehrkunde II (12):665–671
59. Deussen I (1963) Die Entstehung und Bekämpfung der Panik, part 2. Wehrkunde 12 (2):84–90
60. Deussen I (1963) Über Entstehung und Bekämpfung der Panik, part 3. Wehrkunde 12 (3):144–158
61. Djalilov KD (1967) The treatment of cholera in the Kara-Kalpaksky Autonomous SSR of the Uzbek SSR. In: Proceedings of the 4th scientific conference on current problems of infectious pathology, Tashkent, pp 114–116 (in Russian)
62. Djalilov KA (1971) Organization of services to the population during the aftermath of an earthquake. In: The Tashkent earthquake of April 26, 1966. Tashkent, pp 621–626 (in Russian)
63. Davis J (1974) Drought in West Africa. Bull World Meteorological Organization 23 (1):22–29
64. Dimaksian AM (1966) Radiodetection of mudflows. Hydrometeoizdat, Leningrad (in Russian)
65. Dolgushina LD et al (1973) Complex investigation of glaciers and glacial regions. In: Proceedings of the 5th All-Union Glaciological Symposium. Moscow, p 10 (in Russian)
66. Dubos R (1969) Ecology of man. WHO Chron 23 (11):511–516
67. Dubrovsky SL (1967) Problems of current sanitary control in Tashkent during the aftermath of the earthquake. Report delivered at the scientific session on research on the Tashkent earthquake of 1966 and its recurrent tremors. Tashkent, pp 46–47 (in Russian)
68. Duisenov ED (1969) Mudflow protective measures in Zailijsk Alatau. In: Problems of mudflow investigation. Transactions of the Kazakh Hydrometeorological Sci.-Res. Institute, Moscow, vol 33, pp 73–82 (in Russian)
69. Duke CM (1960) The Chilean earthquakes of May 1960. Science 132 (3442):1797–1802
70. Eilers (1962) In Hamburg. Zivilschutz 26 (6):195–200
71. Eitinger L, Grunfeld B (1966) Psychoses among refugees in Norway. Acta Psychiatr Scand 42 (3):315–328
72. Elansky NN (1950) Traumatic toxicosis in mass closed injuries of soft tissues (in Russian). Khirurgija 1:3–7
73. Eldar R (1981) A multi-hospital system for disaster situations. Disasters 5 (2):112–119
74. Eliakis E (1974) Le mort violente par avalanche. Mise au point medico-legale. Med Leg Domage Copp 7 (1):83–87
75. Emelianova VI, Zimnij IM, Lermontov NN, Baranovskaya VA, Rabsh EA (1977) On the state of infectious morbidity in the Pskov region, and the measures for its decrease. In: Epidemiology and prophylaxis of infectious diseases. Leningrad, pp 10–13 (in Russian)

76. Esser AH (1974) Environment and mental health. Sci Med Man 1 (3):181–183
77. Fadeyev AS (1969) Some problems of organization and development of emergency medical aid stations in Tashkent. In: Emergency medical aid. Tashkent, pp 11–14 (in Russian)
78. Fiodorov EK (1978) From description of nature to its design (in Russian). Vopr Filosofii 1:34–49
79. Flaig W (1955) Lawinen. Wiesbaden
80. Flavius Josephus (1900) The Judaean war. St. Petersburg
81. Fleishman SM (1970) Mudflows. Hydrometeoizdat, Leningrad (in Russian)
82. Fleishman SM (1973) The phenomenon of mudflows, and consideration of them in cultivation of mountain territory. In: Fluid exchange and regulation of drainage. Transactions of International Courses of Hydrology, UNESCO, Moscow State University, 4th session, 1972. Moscow, pp 59–68 (in Russian)
83. Fleishman SM (1976) The mudflow. In: Bolshaya Sovetskaya Encyclopedia, 3rd edn, vol 23, p 206. Moscow (in Russian)
84. Fordham IH (1960) Agadir. Postgrad Med J 36 (421):652–657
85. Foster FD (1960) Disaster planning. Hospitals 34 (8):60–64
86. Friesen G (1974) Vancouver Island traffic fatalities. J Trauma 14 (9):791–797
87. Gaffney MP (1973) Public health engineering: pure and political thought. Public Health Eng 6
88. Galanopoulos AG (1960) Tsunamis observed on the coasts of Greece from antiquity to the present time. Am Geofis 13 (3–4):369–386
89. Gankovsky YV (ed) (1966) Pakistan. Guidebook. Moscow (in Russian)
90. Gareyeva MS, Khairulin FY (1968) Skin leishmaniosis in Ashkhabad, and measures for its prophylaxis (in Russian). Zdravookhranenie Turkmenistana 1:37–40
91. Gelshtein EM (1951) Alimentary dystrophy. Etiology and pathogenesis. In: Experience of Soviet medicine in the great patriotic war (1941–1945) vol 28, pp 18–29, Medgiz, Moscow (in Russian)
92. Gelshtein EM, Stotzyk NL (1950) Course and complications in alimentary dystrophy. In: Experience of Soviet medicine in the great patriotic war (1941–1945) vol 28, pp 119–133. Medgiz, Moscow (in Russian)
93. Field Hospital of the German Order of Malta (*Malteser Hilfsdienst*) in the earthquake area of Peru. (1970) Report of the activities of the MHD in Peru, June 10–July 27, 1970. Committee on the Challenges of Modern Society. Disaster Assistance: Earthquake Hazard Reduction, no 9
94. Gilmour AE (1964) Characteristics of tsunamis. Wellington
95. Ginko SS (1965) Catastrophes on riverbanks. In: Conquest of rivers. Hydrometeoizdat, Leningrad, pp 42–54 (in Russian)
96. Glass A (1959) Psychological aspects of disaster. JAMA 171 (2):222–253
97. Goguel J (1965) Traite de tectonique. Paris
98. Golding JS (1974) Changing incidence and pattern of trauma in Jamaica. Br Med J 4 (5940):333–335
99. Golinsky GL, Kallaur TN, Nepesov RD, Lagutochkina KD (1972) The Ashkhabad earthquake of November 15, 1968. In: Earthquakes in the USSR. Nauka, Moscow, pp 50–58 (in Russian)
100. Goldberg DG (1952) Closed injuries of the spine and the spinal marrow. In: Experience of Soviet medicine in the great patriotic war (1941–1945), vol 11, pp 360–382. Medgiz, Moscow (in Russian)
101. Golman SV (1949) Closed trauma of the skull. In: Experience of Soviet medicine in the great patriotic war (1941–1945), vol 4, pp 189–234. Medgiz, Moscow (in Russian)
102. Goriachev AV (1960) The Kamchatka earthquakes of May 4 and June 18, 1959, and the geological conditions of their appearance. Bulletin of the Committee for Seismology, USSR Academy of Science, 11:32–44. Moscow (in Russian)
103. Gorky M, Meyer V (1909) The earthquake in Calabria and Sicily. Capri (in Russian)
104. Gorshkov GP (1970) Prognosis of earthquakes as an important scientific problem. USA Ekonomika Politika Ideologia 6:114–116
105. Grazhul V (1958) Hunger as a biosocial phenomenon. Bolshaya Medizinskaya Encyclopedia, 2nd edn, vol 7, p 948. Moscow (in Russian)

106. Gran MM, Matulsky GS (1926) Typical sanitary conditions in the Jewish village. In: Problems of biology and pathology in Jews. Prakticheskaya Medicina, Leningrad, pp 102–140 (in Russian)
107. Grigorash ZK (1969) Distribution of tsunami in 1927 on the Black Sea. Transactions of the Marine Hydrophysical Institute, USSR Academy of Sciences, 18:113–116 (in Russian)
108. Grigorash ZK, Korneva LA (1972) Oceanographic data on tsunami on the Black Sea at the time of the Turkish earthquake in December, 1939 (in Russian). Okeanologiya 12 (3):417–421
109. Grotian A (1925) Social pathology. Moscow (in Russian) ed 1
110. Guichon DM et al (1975) Bicycle injuries: one year sample in Calgary, Alberta, Canada. J Trauma 15 (6):504–506
111. Guilher A, Fre'caut R (1962) L'onde de tempte de Hamburg et de la côte Allemande de la mer du Nord (16–17 Fevrier 1962). Bull Union Int Secours 38:3–20, Geneve
112. Gussak V, Besedin P (1967) For us and for our grandchildren (in Russian). Pravda Vostoka 118
113. Halloway R (1971) Medical disaster planning in urban areas. NY State J Med 71 (5):591–595
114. Havard JDJ (1979) Mortality from motor vehicle accidents in the 15–24 year age group. WHO Statistics Q 32 (3):225–241
115. Heck NH (1944) Japanese earthquakes. Bull Seismol Soc Am 34 (3):113–136
116. Herz D (1970) Examination of personality trends in people involved in road accidents. Harefuah 80:4
117. Herner B (1966) Br J Int Med 23:40
118. Hodgson JH (1964) Earthquakes and earth structure. Prentice-Hall, Englewood Cliffs, New Jersey
119. Yigiste AK, Yiks UL (1977) Characteristics of the epidemiological process of typhoid in the Estonian SSR. In: Reports delivered at the 3rd Republican Congress of Epidemiologists, Microbiologists, Infectionists, and Hygienists of the Estonian SSR. Tallin, p 32 (in Russian)
120. Ikonnikova LN (1964) The extremely strong tsunami on the Soviet coast of the Pacific Ocean. Transactions of the Far East Sci.-Res. Institute of the Hydrometeorological Institute, Leningrad, 17:69–72 (in Russian)
121. Institut für Schnee- und Lawinenforschung, Davos (1951) Schnee und Lawinen in den Wintern 1936/37 bis 1945/46. Davos
122. Young VR, Scrimshaw N (1971) The physiology of starvation. Sci Am 225 (4):14–21
123. Ivanov AV (1973) Avalanches of Sakhalin and the Kuril Islands. Especially dangerous hydrometeorological phenomena of the Sakhalin region. Yuzhno-Sakhalinsk, pp 154–164 (in Russian)
124. Kadyrov AM, Yusupov KY, Djalalov KD (1973) Comparative epidemiological characteristics of certain intestinal infectious morbidity in Tashkent before and after the earthquake. In: Epidemiological microbiology and clinical-diagnostic infectious pathology in Uzbekistan. Tashkent, pp 31–36 (in Russian)
125. Kahn H (1965) On escalation. New York
126. Kahn H, Wiener AI (1969) The year 2000. A framework for speculation on the next thirty-three years. Macmillan, New York
127. Kamilov FK (1970) Ambulance service during the 1966 Tashkent earthquake. In: Questions concerning the provision of urgent medical aid. Moscow, pp 34–35 (in Russian)
128. Kapovskaya RA, Ilina TS, Myasnikova DE, Tyuneeva GA (1969) Incidence of whooping cough in Tashkent during the period of mass immunization. In: Papers of the Scientific Conference on the Epidemiology of Whooping Cough and "Para-whooping". Meditzina, Moscow, pp 53–58 (in Russian)
129. Karelin L (1969) The earthquake. Moscow (in Russian)
130. Kayumov VG (1967) The impact of an earthquake on the outbreak and course of some endocrine diseases. In: Reports to the scientific session on the findings of research into the results of the Tashkent earthquake. Tashkent, pp 45–46 (in Russian)
131. Karwacki JJ et al (1979) Children in motor vehicles: never too young to die. JAMA 242:26–28, 48–51
132. Kidel AS (1977) Review of seismicity in the Carpatho-Balkans (in Russian). Fisika Zemli 6:119–120

133. Kimura M (1978) The trend of traffic accidents in Tokyo. Proceedings of the Amer Assoc for Automotive Medicine, 22nd Conference, and the International Assoc for Accidents and Traffic Medicine, 7th Conference, Ann Arbor, Michigan, July, pp 25–53
134. Kirnos DP, Rykov AV (1961) Special, quickly functioning seismic apparatus for informing of tsunami approach. Bulletin of the Committee for Seismology, USSR Academy of Sciences 9:56–66, Moscow (in Russian)
135. Klychmuradov K (1974) The Ashkhabad earthquake, 1948 (in Russian). Voen Ist Zh 3:119
136. Kniazhinskaya LA (1974) The population and food supply. Population of countries throughout the world: manual. Statistica, Moscow, pp 440–463 (in Russian)
137. Kolosenko MN (1955) The earthquake on the Ionian islands (in Russian). Priroda 1:128
138. Komarova NG (1974) Mountain ecosystems: principles of their protection and rational use. In: Life of the earth. Moscow State University, vol 10, pp 135–146 (in Russian)
139. Korsunskaya MI (1942) Sanitary provision for evacuated children (in Russian). Gigiene Zdorovye 1 (2):12–17
140. Kort VG (1962) The problem of tsunami (in Russian). Okeanologiya 3 (2):453–456
141. Kotiuminskaya NA, Nevsky MV, Amanova RA, Makarova EI, Aminzade ZM, Yusupova AD (1967) Chronic pathogen-carrying in typhus and paratyphus in the city of Tashkent. In: Proceedings of the 4th Scientific Conference on Topical Problems of Infectious Pathology. Tashkent, pp 19–20 (in Russian)
142. Kovalevskaya KN (1888) Impact of earthquakes on the mental life of man (in Russian). Russkoe Bogatstvo 5 (6):234–242
143. Krayevaya TS (1969) A brief characteristic of mudflow-vulnerable regions of Kamchatka. In: Problems in the study of mudflows. Transactions of the Kazakh Sci.-Res. Institute for Hydrometeorology, vol 33, pp 144–150. Moscow (in Russian)
144. Kukhtinova TI (1966) The earthquakes of Tadzhikistan. Dushanbe (in Russian)
145. Kugelmass IN (1978) The nature of illness in our future society. J Int Assoc Prev Med 5 (1):113–117
146. Kuzin MI (1959) Syndrome following slow crush injury: traumatic toxicosis (in Russian). Khirurgiya 5:16
147. Lachman R, Tatsuoka M, Bank WI (1961) Human behaviour during the tsunami. Research on the Hawaiian disaster explores the consequences of an ambiguous warning system. Science 133 (3462):1405–1409
148. Lane RGT (1971) Seismic activity in man-made reservoirs. Proc Inst Civ Eng 50, Sept. 15–24
149. Lang-Belonogova NS (1952) Hypertensive disease. Experience of Soviet medicine in the great patriotic war (1941–1945), vol 21, pp 175–219. Medgiz, Moscow (in Russian)
150. Llewelyn-Davies R, Macaulay HMC (1966) Hospital planning and administration. Geneva
151. Litvinova VV (1970) Some problems of patients' hospitalization in Tashkent. In: Proceedings of the 44th Scientific Conference of the Tashkent Institute for Professional Advancement of Physicians. Tashkent, pp 21–22 (in Russian)
152. Ljubomirov KS (1975) Inundation in the USSR (in Russian). Vodnye Resursy 2:72–83
153. Lobnovsky AI, Sorokhtin OG, Shemenda AN (1980) Modeling the island arcs deformation, causing appearance of tectonic terraces and of tsunamogenic earthquakes (in Russian). Rep USSR Acad Sci 255 (1):74–77
154. Los VA (1982) Interrelations between man and nature as a global problem (in Russian). Vopr Filosofii 5:128–135
155. Madzhidov NM (1971) Organization of medical provision for the population and urgent problems of antiepidemic services during the aftermath of the 1966 earthquake. In: The Tashkent earthquake of April 26, 1966. Tashkent, pp 620–621 (in Russian)
156. Madzhidov NN, Kariev M, Ablyamitov F (1971) Appearance and clinical course of severe disturbances in cerebral circulation during the Tashkent earthquake. In: The Tashkent earthquake of April 26, 1966. Tashkent, pp 631–635 (in Russian)
157. Madzhidov NM, Kariev MK (1975) Hemorrhage in the brain. Meditzina, Tashkent (in Russian)
158. Magoon OT, Armo NL (1973) Long-term prognosis of floods caused by tsunami for Crescent City, CA, USA. Transactions of SAKHNII: Waves of tsunami, vol 32, pp 162–182. Yuzhno-Sakhalinsk (in Russian)

159. Mahez TF (1955) Medical planning for care of mass casualties in disaster. N Engl Med J 253 (5):205–207
160. Markin VA, Khodakov VG (1971) In the icy world of mountains. Leningrad (in Russian)
161. Mata L (1979) The malnutrition infection complex and its environment factors. Proc Nutr Soc 38 (1):29–40
162. Maksimov NV, Ziabin VV, Barbat YP (1973) Investigation of snow avalanches in the territory of Kirghizia, and the struggle against them. Izvestia Kirgizskogo Geograficheskogo Obshestva 10:96–100
163. Medunin AY (1969) Impact of the scientific-technological revolution on the nature of the earth. Vopr Filosofii 3:23–34
164. Mendelson EI (1978) Hypnosis in the treatment of arterial hypertension disease. Harofeh Haole 5:38–44
165. Mesarovich M, Pestel E, Jerne M (1974) The computer predicts hunger. UNESCO Courier, Aug–Sept, Paris, pp 30–34
166. Mikheyenkov ND (1970) The Azov floods. In: Man and the elements. Leningrad, p 51 (in Russian)
167. Miagkov SM (1967) In: Tushinsky GK (ed) Snow and avalanches in the Khybyns. Moscow (in Russian)
168. Miartin YK, Sudakova RN, Birk KF, Lok EF (1978) Water as a factor in the transmission of dysentery in Estonia. In: Reports delivered at the Symposium of the All-Union Commission on Problems of Epidemiology, Management, Diagnosis, and Prophylaxis of Infectious Diseases. Tallin, pp 54–56 (in Russian)
169. Miesi Hisasi (1961) Nippon Kaiyo Gakkaishi 17 (3):153–156
170. Miln J (1890) Impact of earthquakes on man. Nauka i Zhisn, pp 243–244
171. Medvedev SV (ed) (1968) Seismic zoning of the USSR. Nauka, Moscow
172. Minina L (1972) Tropical cyclones (in Russian). Morskoy Sbornik, p 77
173. Mirimanian KP (1972) The principal problems of protecting nature in mountain regions. In: Proceedings of session of the MSOP Mountain Committee and Scientific Conference on Protection of Mountain Landscapes, June 21–28, 1971, Yerevan, pp 17–27 (in Russian)
174. Misra RP (1978) Nutrition and health in India, 1950–2000 AD. J Hum Evol 7 (1):85–93
175. Montandon F (1959) Quelle est la moyenne annualle des morts causee par la tremblement de terres? Revue pour l'etude des calamites. Bull Union Int Secours 36:64–65
176. Mossakovskaya IA (1972) Engineering-geological investigations in the region of the Serez lake. In: Problems of engineering geology of Tadzhikistan. Donim, Dushanbe, pp 125–131 (in Russian)
177. Mstislavsky PS (1972) Hunger. Bolshaya Sovetskaya Encyclopedia, 3rd edn, vol 7, pp 83–84 (in Russian)
178. Mullen JT (1974) The magnitude of the problem of trauma. J Trauma 14 (12):1070–1072
179. Murty TS, Henry RF (1973) Some investigations of tsunami behaviour on the western Canadian coast. Transactions of SAKHNII: Waves of tsunami, vol 32, pp 110–128. Yuzhno-Sakhalinsk
180. Murzayev E (1961) Central Asia. Moscow (in Russian)
181. Nagi NA, Al-Dubooni HM (1977) Severe protein energy malnutrition in Iraq and its effect on immunity reactions. J Trop Med Hyg 80 (4):78–82
182. Napetvaridze SG (1973) Some problems of engineering seismology. Meznierebe, Tbilisi (in Russian)
183. Naumov IN (1973) The problem of food provision in China. Moscow (in Russian)
184. Nazarov AG, Shakhsuvarijan LV, Piruzian SA, Zakarian VA (1973) Microseismic investigation of the Zangezursk earthquake. In: Results of complex investigation of the Zangezursk earthquake. Armenian SSR Academy of Science, Yerevan, pp 22–53 (in Russian)
185. Negrobov AI (1928) Impact of war on the everyday domestic conditions and the public health situation in the countries involved (in Russian). Profilakticheskaya Meditzina 2:70
186. New York Times (1982) Los Angeles is preparing for the possible earthquake. Cited in Krug 270:44
187. Novograblenov P (1923) The earthquake in Ust-Kamchatsk, April 14, 1923. Poliarnaya Zvezda 96

188. Kotchari, Bchabcha, Kchanolkaz (1958) Nuclear explosions. Inostrannaya Literatura, Moscow (in Russian)
189. Orazymbetov NO, Serdiukov MM, Shashin SA (1960) The Ashkhabad earthquake 1948 (an engineering analysis of the consequences). Moscow (in Russian)
190. Ovchinnikov V (1966) Information (in Russian). Sovetskaya Rossiya 110
191. Ovezov AO, Chairulin FY (1969) Maintenance of adequate facilities in relation to cutaneous leishmaniasis in Ashkhabad. In: Proceedings of 3rd conference on leishmaniasis and other contagious tropical diseases among the people of Central Asia and the Trans-Caucasian region. Moscow, pp 132–133 (in Russian)
192. Parrack DW (1978) Famine symposium: ecosystems and famine. Ecol Food Nutr 1:17–21
193. Parrisch HM, Baker AS, Bischop F (1964) Epidemiology in public health planning for natural disasters. Public Health Rep 79 (10):863–867
194. Petrova I, Zhitlovsky K (1927) In the face of a new danger: Lessons of the 1926 flood. Kazan (in Russian)
195. Petrova NS, Kamilov FK (1969) The impact of the Tashkent earthquake on the neurovascular systems of the inhabitants of Tashkent. In: Reports of the first aid service. Tashkent, pp 98–100 (in Russian)
196. Podyapolsky P (1928) The significance of sleep during an earthquake (in Russian). Klin Zh Saratovskogo Univ 1 (5):39–42
197. Pokrovskaya VI (1967) The water factor in the epidemiology of tularemia in the Novgorod region (in Russian). Pasteur Inst Epidemiol Microbiol Leningrad 31:57–61
198. Pokrovsky VI, Tutelian VA (1982) Ergotism as the companion of natural disasters (in Russian). Terapeut Arkh 9:108–110
199. Poniavin ID (1968) The waves of tsunami. Leningrad (in Russian)
200. Popov VI (1932) The flood in DVK. Blagoveshchensk (in Russian)
201. Popov GI (1961) On the conditions for tsunami formation. Bulletin of Commission for Seismology, USSR Academy of Science, vol 9, pp 7–22. Moscow (in Russian)
202. Popovic M, Petrovic D (1964) After the earthquake. Lancet 2 (7370):1169–1171
203. Pratt D (1965) Casualty handling in nuclear war. Mil Rev Sept: 78–84
204. Rayevskaya NT, Djamalova ZM, Khanakjan EGm Khodjibayeva RK (1971) Some peculiarities in the course of pregnancy and delivery in Tashkent women during the earthquake. In: The Tashkent earthquake of April 26, 1966. Tashkent, pp 644–645 (in Russian)
205. Rai IA (1967) The flood along the lower Danube. Meteorologiya i Hydrologiya 9:74–76
206. Rayushkin BV (1967) Typhoid epidemiology and prophylaxis in the Alma-Ata region. In: Proceedings of the 4th Scientific Conference on Topical Problems in Infectious Pathology, Tashkent, pp 244–246 (in Russian)
207. Ravenstein EG (1885/1889) The laws of migration. J R Statist Soc vols 48 and 52
208. Report of the Krakatoa Committee of the Royal Society (1888) London
209. Richter ED (1979) Potential years of life lost in motor vehicle crashes in Israel. An epidemiological analysis. Int J Epidemiol 8 (4):383–388
210. Riemersma JBJ (1979) Perception in traffic. Urban Ecol 4 (2):139–149
211. Ryzhikov IE (1967) Rabbit fever in some regions of northwestern Russia during the war (1942–1943). In: Rabbit fever in the northwest RSFSR. Pasteur Inst Epidemiol Microbiol Leningrad (in Russian)
212. Riznichenko YV (1969) Topics set for research in seismic progression. In: Proceedings of the 1st All-Union Symposium on Seismic Regimes, December 12–17, 1966, Dushanbe, pp 3–13 (in Russian)
213. Rothe JP (1946) Seismes et volcans. Presses Universitaires, Paris, pp 31–32
214. Rothe JP (1961) Les seismes de Chili, revue pour l'etudes des calamites. Bull Union Int Secours 37:3–14
215. Rousseau P (1961) Les tremblements. Paris
216. Rudashev E, Yashchenko N (1969) Sanitary-chemical and sanitary-bacteriological characteristics of the Narym basin waters. In: Problems of regional epidemiology and hygiene, Kirgistan. Frunze (in Russian)
217. Rustanovich DN (1967) Seismicity of territory in Turkmen SSR, and the Ashkhabad earthquake of 1948, 12th edn. Moscow (in Russian)

218. Savarensky EF, Tishchenko VG, Sviatlovsky AE, Dobrovolsky AD, Zhivago AV (1958) Tsunami of the 4–5 November 1952. Bulletin of the Committee for Seismology, USSR Academy of Science, vol 4. Moscow (in Russian)
219. Savarensky EF (1977) Development of Soviet seismology over 60 years (1917–1977) (in Russian). Fizika Zemli 12:87–97
220. Shafranskaya KD (1967) Study of man in extreme conditions. In: Man and society, vol 2, pp 226–235. Leningrad University (in Russian)
221. Shamov VN, Ryzhkov SV, Kopospv ES (1962) The problems of treating acute renal insufficiency by means of the artificial kidney device. Voen Med Zh 11
222. Sharipov MK, Kaplunova MS, Smirnova TG, Kaplunova GI (1967) Dysentery morbidity in the Uzbek SSR. In: Proceedings of the 4th Scientific Conference on Topical Problems of Infectious Pathology, Tashkent, pp 61–62 (in Russian)
223. Shcherba ML (1951) Pneumonia as a complication of injuries of other localization. In: Experience of Soviet medicine in the great patriotic war (1941–1945). Medgiz, Moscow 29:62–78 (in Russian)
224. Shepard F (1948) Submarine geology. New York
225. Shepard FP, Macdonald GA, Cox DC (1950) The tsunami of April 1, 1946. Bull Scripps Inst Oceanogr 5
226. Shipunov FY (1969) Will the mountains live? (in Russian) Priroda 9:82–90
227. Selim R (1980) The 1980s. A decade of hunger. Futures 14 (2):323
228. Selya RM (1980) Death due to accidents in Taiwan: a possible indicator of development. Soc Sci Med 14 (4):361–367
229. Selye H (1952) The story of the adaptation syndromes (series of informal, illustrated lectures). Montreal, Canada
230. Sencer DJ, Foege WH, Kaiser RL, Feldman RA (1976) Epidemiological assessment of earthquake relief, Guatemala, February 4–March 10, 1976. Memorandum, Washington, April 26
231. Symson T (1928) Psychic and psychotic reactions to earthquakes in adults and children. Transactions of the Psychiatric Clinic of Moscow State University, 3:419–431 (in Russian)
232. Sokolov AN, Grilikhes IA, Kolerov VP (1944) Health security in transport. In: Twenty-five years of Soviet health security services. Gosmedizdat, Moscow, pp 262–272 (in Russian)
233. Solovjov SL, Tarakanov RZ, Solovjova ON, Oskorbin LS, Go Chin Nam (1967) Earthquakes and tsunamis. Atlas of the Sakhalin region. Moscow, pp 41–44 (in Russian)
234. Solovjev SL (1968) The problems of tsunami and their significance for Kamchatka and the Kuril Islands. In: Problems of tsunami. Moscow, pp 7–50 (in Russian)
235. Solovjov SL, Go Chin Nam (1974) Catalogue of tsunami on the western coast of the Pacific Ocean. Nauka, Moscow (in Russian)
236. Solovjov SL (1978) Tsunami. In: Bolshaya Sovetskaya Encyclopedia, 3rd edn, vol 28, p 605 (in Russian)
237. Somogyi JC (1979) Nutritional problems in developing and industrial countries, and possibilities for their solution. Solut Nutr Probl: Contrib Prod, Distrib and Nutr Symp. Zürich, 1978. Basel
238. Sorochinsky MA (1970) Avalanches and snow storms, winter 1969/1970. In: Man and the elements. Hydrometeoizdat, Leningrad, pp 38–40 (in Russian)
239. Sosnitsky VI, Nekrasova LI (1967) Epidemiology of tularemia in the Nenetzk National District of the Arkhangelsk region. In: Tularemia in the northwest RSFSR. Pasteur Inst Epidemiol Microbiol Leningrad 31:83–91 (in Russian)
240. Sound PW (1964) Alaskan earthquakes. Rev Union Int Secours 2:40–69
241. Anonymous (1964) Guidebook for prognosis and control of snow avalanches. Progress, Moscow (in Russian)
242. Stallones RA (1972) Environment, ecology and epidemiology. WHO Chron 26 (11):498–502
243. Stavissky YS (1972) Catastrophes in mountains. In: Man and the elements. Hydrometeoizdat, Leningrad, p 168 (in Russian)
244. Stockle B (1974) Christliche Verantwortung und Umweltfragen. Stimmen der Zeit 12:836
245. Stolpyansky N (1926) The inundation in Leningrad on September 23, 1924. Kubuch, Leningrad (in Russian)

246. Takahasi R (1951) An estimate of future tsunami damage along the Pacific coast of Japan. Bull Earthqu Res Inst (Tokyo University) 29 (1):71–95
247. Tarasevich LA (1922) Epidemics of recent years in Russia (in Russian). Obshestvenniy Vrach 1:43–50
248. Tazieff H (1962) Quand la terre tremble. Paris
249. Timofeyev N (1958) Psychic changes during hunger. Bolshaya Meditzinskaya Encyclopedia, 2nd edn, vol 7, p 961 (in Russian)
250. Tushinsky GK, Fleishman SM (1972) Avalanche and mudflow risk information service in the USSR. In: Man and the elements. Hydrometeoizdat, Leningrad, pp 170–171 (in Russian)
251. Tushinsky GK (1973) Calculation of avalanche danger in construction design. In: Fluid exchange and regulation of drainage. Studies of International Advanced Courses for Hydrology, UNESCO, Moscow State University, 4th session, 1972. Moscow, pp 69–80 (in Russian)
252. Umakhanov MSI (1970) On the tasks of the regional party organization in light of the implementation of the CC CPSU regulation and the decision of the Soviet of Ministers of the USSR on measures of help to the Daghestan Autonomous SSR in elimination of the earthquake consequences (in Russian). Daghestanskaya Pravda 136, July 12
253. Umidova ZI, Aripdzhanov AA, Korolev GP, Timbekova ZK, Mukhamedzhina AG, Burleva SM (1968) Course of heart attacks during the Tashkent earthquake, 1966–1967 (in Russian). Kardiologiya 2:25–27
254. Urazbayev MT, Raskazovsky VT, Rashidov TR et al (1971) Analysis of seismic impact on buildings. In: The Tashkent earthquake, 1966. Tashkent, pp 470–527 (in Russian)
255. Vinogradov YV (1969) Formation of mudflows and methods of calculating them. In: Problems of mudflow studies. Transactions of the Kazakh Hydrometeorological Institute 33:5–29 (in Russian)
256. Vakhula IA (1978) Epidemiology and prophylaxis of intestinal infections. In: Reports delivered at Symposium of All-Union Commission on the Problems of Epidemiology, Management, Diagnosis, and Prophylaxis of Infectious Diseases. Tallin, pp 61–63 (in Russian)
257. Varshavsky S, Rest B (1978) A ticket for all eternity. Lenizdat, Leningrad, p 311 (in Russian)
258. Vishnevsky AA, Shraiber MI (1965) Military field surgery. Meditzina, Moscow (in Russian)
259. Vlodavetz VI (1956) On tsunami connected with volcanic eruptions. Bulletin of the Committee for Seismology, USSR Academy of Science 2:27–30 (in Russian)
260. Wagner EA, Firsov VD, Chereshnev VA, Bruns VA et al. (1980) Clinical course, diagnosis and treatment of a grave combined thoracic injury (in Russian). Sovetskaya Meditzina 10:84–85
261. Waldner R (1974) Wie der Arzt im Katastrophenfall vorgehen muß. Zivilschutz 3:86–87
262. Ward B, Dubos R (1972) Only one earth. New York
263. Watanabe K, Oshima Y, Yshizaka T, Araki H, Miyamoto T, Hirose S (1967) Weather and asthma in Japan. Biometeorology 2 (1):28
264. Webre AL, Liss PH (1974) The age of cataclysm. New York
265. Wortraich B, Baat L (1971) Presentation of medical information about sick drivers to the traffic board. Harefuah 80:90–91
266. Anonymous (1969) Psychophysiological causes of traffic accidents. WHO Chron 23 (5):207–213
267. Zabirov RD (1968) International symposium on snow avalanches and ice avalanches (in Russian). Izvestia Kirgizskogo Geograficheskogo Obsbestva 7:84–89
268. Zalogin BS, Rodionov NA (1969) The mouth regions of rivers in the USSR. Moscow
269. Zilper ZZ, Savitskaya LA (1968) Traumas and myocardial infarctions as direct consequences of the Tashkent earthquake. In: Anthology of material from the 3rd Conference of Young Scientists of the Tashkent Medical Institute. Tashkent, pp 314–315 (in Russian)
270. Solomons NW, Butte NA (1978) A view of the medical and nutritional consequences of the earthquake in Guatemala. Public Health Rep 93 (2):161–169
271. Tourarinson S (1974) Life on the volcano. UNESCO Courier, February, pp 4–8
272. Nozdriakov AP (1981) Man – road – car (in Russian). Sociologicheskie Issledovania 3:113–117
273. Toffler A (1980) The third wave. William Morrow, New York
274. Friedle H, Ramharter F (1980) Gesundheitsstatistik 1979 (part 1). Statist Nahr 35 (11):640–642
275. TASS (1967) Natural disasters and health security, vol 1:43,53,80 (in Russian)
276. Za Rubezhom (1970) Moscow, January 30 – February 5, p 27 (in Russian)

277. TzGIAL USSR 1288 (13)16, pp 95–96
278. TzGIAL USSR 1276 (25)48, p 660
279. Dagestanskaya Pravda (1970) May 21, no 117
280. USSR Ministry of Health Archives no 7a, op 356, pp 59–113, 125
281. TASS (1966) Natural disasters and health security, no 221, vol 3, p 69 (in Russian)
282. TASS (1968) Natural disasters and health security, no 275, vol 2, p 262 (in Russian)
283. Central State October Revolution Archives file 9501, op 1, unit 114, p 9
284. Central State October Revolution Archives unit 190, pp 30, 32, 41–43, 222
285. Central State October Revolution Archives unit 261, p 10
286. TASS materials
287. Uzbek SSR Ministry of Health (Aripov U) report to the USSR Ministry of Health (1966)
288. USSR Ministry of Health Archives no 7a, op 356, unit 39, pp 59, 113
289. USSR Ministry of Health Archives op 5a, unit 175
290. USSR Ministry of Health (1950) Protocol no 33 of Collegial Meeting, July 18, pp 94, 95, 96
291. USSR Ministry of Health Archives op 391, unit 829, p 223
292. October Revolution State Archives, Leningrad region, 104, op 1, archive unit 122, pp 69, 83, 92
293. USSR Ministry of Health, op 211a, archive unit 279
294. State Archives of the October Revolution, Legingrad region, f 4301, op 1, archive unit 1769, pp 303, 304
295. State Archives of the October Revolution, Leningrad region, op 1, archive unit 85, p 99
296. State Archives of the October Revolution, Leningrad region, f 7, op 1, rep 257, p 12
297. Yevgeny Gabovich, citing Bu Yong Ming (1982) China: Population, Environment, Resources. Russkaya Mysl no 3437, Nov 4, p 5 (in Russian)
298. World Health Organization Chronicle (1977) vol 25, no 6, p 266
299. TASS (1967) Natural disasters and health security, no 277, vol 3, pp 161, 172 (in Russian)
300. TASS (1967) Natural disasters and health security, no 277, vol 1, pp 55, 92 (in Russian)
301. TASS (1967) Natural disasters and health security, vol 3, pp 49, 51–52, 93 (in Russian)
302. Cobo J (1970) Grave days in Peru. Novoye Vremia, no 25, July 19, p 26 (in Russian)
303. Medical Reference Journal, Moscow (1969) no 2, ch 16, p 28 (in Russian)
304. Volodicheva NA (1970)
305. Borba (1970) Yugoslavia, April 17
306. Severskij IV et al (1969)
307. October Revolution Central Archives, f 1064, op 3, archive unit 21, pp 1–4
308. October Revolution Central Archives, f 1064, op 3, archive unit 1, pp 14–17
309. October Revolution Central Archives, f 1064, op 3, archive unit 21, p 2
310. October Revolution Archives of Socialist Construction, Leningrad region, f 5876, op 5–96, p 61
311. October Revolution Archives of Socialist Construction, Leningrad region, f 4301, op 1/858, p 21
312. October Revolution Archives of Socialist Construction, Leningrad region, f 4301, op 1/642
313. Bolshaya Sovetskaya Entzyklopedija (1972) 3rd edn. vol 9, p 1036
314. World History 3rd edn (1973) Moscow, vol 14, p 306
315. October Revolution Archives of Socialist Construction, Leningrad region, f 9156, op 4/93, p 19
316. October Revolution Archives of Socialist Construction, Leningrad region, f 9156, op 4/94
317. October Revolution Archives of Socialist Construction, Leningrad region, f 9156, op 4/91, pp 67, 69
318. October Revolution Archives of Socialist Construction, Leningrad region, f 9156, op 4/111, p 146
319. Statistical Guidebook of the Populations Public Health Conditions during the years of the Great Patriotic War. Moscow, Library of the Dept for Medical Statistics of the USSR Health Ministry, no 227 (in Russian)
320. Shitnikova ZZ Brief review of the sanitary situation in Leningrad during the war, 1941–1945. Central October Revolution State Archives of the USSR, f 8009, archive unit 1985, p 36 (in Russian)
321. Central October Revolution State Archives of the USSR, op 6, archive unit 1984, p 32

322. Central October Revolution State Archives of the USSR, f 9156, op 4/95, p 24
323. Central State Archives of the USSR's People's Husbandry, f 1884, op 331, archive unit 3514, pp 7–9
324. Central State Archives of the USSR's People's Husbandry, f 1884, op 31, archive unit 3520, pp 1–3
325. USSR Defense Ministry Archives, f 217, op 1250/66, pp 33–35
326. October Revolution Archives of Socialist Construction, Leningrad region, f 330, op 1, archive unit 154
327. TASS (1966) Natural disasters and health security, no 221, p 221 (in Russian) vol 2
328. October Revolution State Archives of the USSR, f 9501, op 1, archive unit 190, p 30
329. October Revolution State Archives of the USSR, f 9501, op 1, archive unit 190, pp 41–43
330. Archives of the USSR Health Ministry, 7a, op 356, pp 124–125, 31
331. Archives of the USSR Health Ministry, op 5a, archive unit 175, pp 61–63, 77
332. Archives of the USSR Health Ministry, op 5a, archive unit 175, pp 66, 88
333. Archives of the USSR Health Ministry, no 1945, op 219a/65, pp 1–3
334. Vishnevsky AA. Archives of the USSR Health Ministry, no 7a, op 356, p 17
335. October Revolution State Archives of the USSR, f 4301, op 1, archive unit 1781, p 46
336. Archives of the USSR Ministry of Health, no 7a, op 356, pp 91–93
337. Archives of the USSR Ministry of Health, no 7a, op 356, p 6
338. Pravda, October 9, 1948
339. Pravda Vostoka. Tashkent, June 7, 1966, no 126
340. October Revolution Central State Archives, f 8009, op 1, archive unit 432, pp 99, 110
341. October Revolution Central State Archives, f 8009, op 1, archive unit 430, pp 39–40, 43, 171
342. Archives of the USSR Health Ministry, op 5a, archive unit 132, pp 96–99, 131
343. Materials of the Voroshilovgrad Hospital No. 4, 1964
344. October Revolution State Archives of Socialist Construction, Leningrad region, f 9156, op 4/116
345. October Revolution State Archives of Socialist Construction, Leningrad region, f 9156, op 4/134, pp 3–4
346. Materials for the brief report on activities of the Russian Federal Republic's Commissariat of Health (1943), p 14
347. USSR Ministry of Health Archives, no 7a, op 356, p 143
348. Nasha Strana, no 3432, January 16, 1983, p 6, Tel Aviv
349. USSR Ministry of Health Archives, no 7a, op 356
350. Salisbury HA The 900-day siege of Leningrad, 1969, New York
351. San Francisco and Vicinity 1976. Frisco Books
352. USSR Ministry of Health Archives, op 211a, archive unit 279. Scientific–Methodological Bureau of Public Health Statistics of the Russian Soviet Federal Socialist Republic
353. Zaria Vostoka (1968) no 93, no 98
354. Pravda Vostoka (1967) no 101–105

GPSR Compliance

The European Union's (EU) General Product Safety Regulation (GPSR) is a set of rules that requires consumer products to be safe and our obligations to ensure this.

If you have any concerns about our products, you can contact us on ProductSafety@springernature.com

In case Publisher is established outside the EU, the EU authorized representative is:

Springer Nature Customer Service Center GmbH
Europaplatz 3
69115 Heidelberg, Germany

Batch number: 10704763

Printed by Printforce, the Netherlands